PRAISE FOR *GET WELL SOON*

"Get Well Soon *is a wise and tender, necessary book, filled with a truth born of searing experience. The memoir charts one man's journey through intractable long-term illness, but it would be infinitely recognisable to anyone whose certainties have been shattered and who has had to rebuild… The book is just so lovely.*"

A.L. Kennedy

"*A fascinating and moving story of one man's attempts to regain his health and vitality. I enjoyed the love and resilience that underpin the struggles and searching.*"

Cathy Rentzenbrink

"*An intelligent, incisive exploration of the cures trotted out to treat the 21st century's most insidious malaise. And no, it's not all in your head.*"

Meg Rosoff

GET WELL SOON

Adventures in Alternative Healthcare

Nick Duerden

BLOOMSBURY

LONDON · OXFORD · NEW YORK · NEW DELHI · SYDNEY

Green Tree
An imprint of Bloomsbury Publishing Plc

50 Bedford Square	1385 Broadway
London	New York
WC1B 3DP	NY 10018
UK	USA

www.bloomsbury.com

First published 2018

British Library Cataloguing-in-Publication Data
A catalogue record for this book is available from the British Library.

Library of Congress Cataloguing-in-Publication data has been applied for.

ISBN: Print: 978-1-4729-5048-2
ePDF: 978-1-4729-5047-5
ePub: 978-1-4729-5049-9

2 4 6 8 10 9 7 5 3 1

Typeset in Fournier by Deanta Global Publishing Services, Chennai, India
Printed and bound in Great Britain by CPI Group (UK) Ltd,
Croydon, CR0 4YY

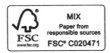

For Elena, of course

'I don't feel well.' Woody Allen, *Hannah and Her Sisters*

Part One

NO CURE

Prologue

One early spring morning, three years into what I laughably hope will prove the defining illness of my life, I find myself sitting opposite a woman in her sun-drenched suburban living room as she tells me about the rise and rise of alternative therapy. She is part of that rise, an independent therapist who mixes elements of hypnotherapy with the purportedly beneficial convergence of mind, consciousness and thought. I nod earnestly as she talks, and I say 'right', and 'okay', and 'yes'. But I cannot quite get a foothold into what it is she, or it, actually does, how it helps, or how I can teach myself to do it for general betterment. But she is nice, and I find I want to make the effort. She tells me that she brings her teaching to bear on an array of modern health issues. Her website reports considerable success. Everything she says makes sense, the words sliding together in neat little rows like agreeable dominoes whose dots align. But when I read up on it later, I'm still a little lost, the sensation uncomfortably redolent of all those lessons at school in which I was doomed to fail.

For example. These principles she expounds upon, when employed successfully, point towards a pre-existing logic that explains human experience. 'Right,' I think. 'Okay.' It represents a renaissance of the mind based on universal constants that uncover our innate natural resilience. 'Yes,' I agree. But then I think: 'Huh?'

I need to understand all this, at root level, because if I do maybe I will become better, and I am not better yet. This is all comparatively new territory for me, territory I thought I would never have to map, but I do, and so here I am. I am still very much a beginner in all this, with much to learn. I'm feeling my way through.

I know, at least, why I'm here talking to the nice lady who is fundamentally not, by anybody's standards, a doctor. I was unwell for ages, a long time. I didn't get better. Because my symptoms were vague, almost elliptical, and didn't show up on X-rays or in blood tests, they were difficult to confirm, to correctly diagnose or act upon. I fell through NHS cracks, and because I did not meet the required criteria for further intervention, I was on my own. I had tried the prescriptions, and all the pills. I had been referred to specialists who developed sudden itches in my presence, and scratched their heads. But then mine was the kind of condition that came with multiple theories attached, and little in the way of a standard pathology. All I really knew of it was this: that the starting point had been a virus. The virus had caused my blood vessels to constrict, and my blood flow to diminish. My adrenal response skyrocketed. My mitochondria had become dysfunctional. I crashed.

Naturally, I comprehended very little of this, but the reading I did into it suggested I was in good company: millions of people were experiencing negative adrenal responses too, and dysfunctions of their mitochondrias, and so were presumably feeling much like I was, like a tuning fork struck hard, the vibrations continuing to ring through my body almost constantly. In such a state, life as I had known it was impossible to sustain.

The abnormal state endured, displaying impressive staying power. It was at the point I feared it might come to define me for ever that I decided to do something that, for me, was radical, and cross the Rubicon from one form of medicine which I didn't much understand but had unquestioning faith in, to another which seemed to me the stuff of parody, patchouli-scented and hung suspended in a purple haze. But people, strangers, said it worked, and that would do because it had to. Scepticism, on which I had previously thrived, no longer served my best interests. I had to find another way.

Initially I had a problem with this because surely there wasn't another way? In my life, there had only ever been the GP, whose advice over the years I had sought infrequently. If she was now not in a position to help me out, what then? The last time I saw her on this matter, her farewell words to me were ominous ones: good luck.

Don't we make our own luck?

One

A wise man – not Confucius, somebody else – once said that we spend the first 40 years of our lives trying to kill ourselves, and the next 40 trying to stay alive.

I spent the first 40 of mine in a perpetual rush. Everything I did I did in a kind of fast-forward, as if in a race towards some imagined finish line, a gold medal to the winner. I ran when I could have walked, and when I walked, I did so briskly, much faster than my wife, who lagged leisurely behind. I worked a lot, all the time, often too much, evenings, weekends, birthdays, and thrilled to every deadline met. I rarely relaxed, but then who needs to relax? In my downtime, I went out for fast walks, for bike rides, shopping, to see friends. I read books, many books, the pile never diminishing because I never stopped buying more. I was always very aware of the pile, earmarking the next book to read before finishing the current one, and earmarking the one after that, too. In the pool, even though I have never been a strong swimmer, always needing to catch my breath after the completion of each length, I would nevertheless try to swim faster than the person in the next lane. Just for fun, a little harmless competition. I was victorious at least 80 per cent of the time, the person I had beaten completely unaware. On my bike, I would instinctively pedal as fast as I could go, faster still when approaching traffic lights, slipping through amber with great satisfaction. If a journey required 20 minutes, I'd complete it in 12, 13; *10* if I went flat out, which I often did. I travelled for work, and once off the aeroplane would always overtake every other passenger in my path, the first to passport control, to the cab rank. At the hotel, a quick shower and then out into the unfamiliar city to ensure I got to know it as thoroughly as one could in 48, 72 hours, strolling its streets, getting happily lost, new adventures around every corner. I was always tired, always complaining about it, but it never seemed to matter, not really. I slept well, I recovered, and ploughed on. After the children were born, they passed on every germ that came their way, and so I was perpetually sniffing, drowsy, battling fevers, tonsillitis and, more than once, worms. Each weekend, we'd head into town somewhere, browsing the city's streets and parks and zoos and markets, rain or shine, taking full advantage of everything the capital had to offer. My life was full, and full of challenge. It took plenty out of me, but life takes plenty out of everybody. I loved it.

But then, incrementally enough to ultimately take me unawares, it all became a bit too much, and though I couldn't know it, and wouldn't have accepted it even if I had known it, things were approaching an emphatic full stop. In blissful ignorance, I was doing things that I would not be able to do again for some considerable time. I took my last long cycle ride in the country, I forget where exactly, someplace south, near Devon, my wife by my side, the girls strapped into child seats behind us, eight miles through pretty, winding lanes, then off-road through woodland, uphill to where the view was, as the leaflet had promised, breathtaking.

'Look, girls. Look at the view.'

They were fast asleep, heads lolling at 45-degree angles.

I took my last flight, 11 hours west, which had been an all too regular journey for me, but this time with the added novelty of First Class, as if the universe was wise to what was lurking in my immediate future and was seeing me off for the final time in style.

'More champagne, sir?'

It was 10 o'clock on a damp Tuesday morning. 'Why not?'

I took my last daily swim, enjoying the thrill of the freezing water that, one length in, turned out not to be freezing at all. My last wallow in the jacuzzi with its strange sulphuric smell, its water slick, almost oily, and the familiar horror when it shot up my nose and slid down the back of my throat to settle queasily in my stomach.

My last restaurant meal with friends, the last time I'd be able to drink wine, the last time, even, I would be able to walk to the corner shop without thinking about it, as if it, the very action of walking, were the most natural thing in the world.

In February 2009, I had been in America for work, and shared a four-hour car journey with someone who said they really should be at home, in bed, convalescing. He had had flu, he told me, a more severe strain than he had ever experienced. People were saying that it had originated in southern California and northern Mexico, and that it might have come from birds, always a bad sign. He was over the worst of it now, but still, *boy*, it was terrible. He had felt awful, a carcass. He laughed as he said this, and so, politely, I laughed back. Later, in the evening, we shared another four-hour journey back to the hotel, and I counted every sneeze that caught him unawares, every cough he failed to catch.

The following day was a long one, in which I was required to watch musicians walk on a red carpet I myself was not permitted on, and it culminated in food, drink and a hot bath to compound the jet lag and offer up the possibility of sleep.

I awoke the morning after, and went across the road to a Starbucks for breakfast. It was in the queue, already full with office workers in bright white trainers, that I began to feel strange, dizzy, disoriented, the simple placing of one foot in front of the other suddenly a challenge as mental as it was physical. I purchased my coffee and croissant, and sat by the window, book in hand. But I could not focus on the words on the page. My appetite evaporated. Moments later I was stumbling back across the road to the hotel, the urge to lie down a powerful one. I sat on my bed, then lay across it, then got bored, then went out, convinced all I needed was some fresh air. The walk to Book Soup took 20 minutes, much of it up a gradual incline. It felt like forever. Once there, I couldn't read the letters on the spines, my vision blurred. I sat for a few moments on the small stepladder people used to access the higher shelves. Somebody asked if I was okay. 'You don't look well, buddy.' I left the shop, stumbling back outside. I needed a cab, but there were none. The walk back was long.

In my room, things were happening fast. I was hot and cold and heavy. I couldn't move. I tried to sleep, in vain. My flight home was in nine hours. I needed to pack. The phone rang. I couldn't reach it. It rang again, and this time I could. It was front desk telling me that I should have checked out by now. I must have slept, after all. Front desk said that I was facing a $50 surcharge unless I vacated in the next quarter hour. I remained in bed another two hours, the sheets soaked in my sweat, and twisted beneath me. Shortly after one, I stumbled downstairs, lightheaded and feverish. The receptionist called a doctor, and handed me the phone. The doctor was happy to come and see me right away, he said. He sounded eager. His callout fee was $350.

'I'll be fine,' I told him.

'*Don't hang up!*' he shouted. I was taken aback by the shouting; I hadn't intended to hang up on him. 'Okay,' he said, 'how about $290?' I thanked him all the same. 'Okay, *okay.*' He was sounding exasperated now. '$250, low as I can go.'

I wasn't used to haggling for medical care, and explained that I didn't think I really needed it. It was flu, presumably the same flu the man in the car had had, the one from birds. I told him again I'd be fine. I would go and see my GP as soon as I got home. The doctor, his voice resigned now, recommended some medicine, 'the strongest over-the-counter available', and wished me a safe flight.

The fever ratcheted up. I could not stand or sit. Everything itched and ached. I thought I might pass out. A cab came. The nearest pharmacy, I said, then the airport. The small print on the box said one capsule every four hours, do not exceed the stated dose. Fearful I would be too ill to be permitted to board the plane, I swallowed two.

The next two weeks were a blur, but during this time I was the illest I had been. Almost no food at all, and I only took water when Elena, my wife, insisted on it. Days and nights passed, all of them jumbled together. One night, shortly before dawn, I found myself in the shower, curled up on the floor, teeth chattering furiously, and wondered how I had got there. I had never been delirious before. It was an almost fun sensation. But not quite.

I got better, eventually, the virus relegated to little more than a war wound I carried with me the way people, stereo-typically men, do. If I never felt quite as good as I had before it, as fit and healthy and hale, then this was a small factor I chose not to dwell on. I was getting older, after all, so this was presumably merely a symptom of that most inescapable of fates. After another year of frequent colds, nothing serious, and plenty of worms, I was hit by flu again, a milder strain this time, but it still wiped out all of Christmas and the New Year celebrations. It wasn't until the second week of January that I felt strong enough to venture out, and I can still remember the novelty of being in the crisp open air amid the bustle of care-less shoppers, each as impatient as I always had been to reach their destination ahead of time, to steal back seconds from the clock. Right now, I didn't feel like one of them. Instead, I was a caricature of an old man, taking my time, counting my footsteps. Halfway to the shopping centre, I saw a public bench I had never previously noticed. An elderly lady was sitting at one end, nosing through her plastic shopping bags. For a few moments I sat self-consciously alongside her, then texted a friend about my plight. She joked that I was indeed an old man now, that I would never be the same again.

A few days later, health restored, that most humdrum of miracles, I resumed my daily routine. Mid-morning, I stopped work and went for a swim. It felt good to be back, racing unwitting strangers, and winning. Within 24 hours, the flu symptoms returned. Frustrated, I rested for a few more days. Then, better again, I returned to the pool. The next morning, I could not get out of bed.

My legs began to feel the strain of cycling, and whenever I attempted, because of course I always did, to speed up and slip through on amber, thighs pumping like pistons, I paid the price for it afterwards, my muscles on fire, and experiencing a level of physical exhaustion that left me reeling. Sprawled out on the sofa was the only recovery position.

I was blithe about it, unconcerned. I tried to get on with life as normal, but the cold and flu symptoms, the shocking bursts of total wipeout, refused to let me. I stopped swimming, my trunks hanging forlorn and ignored on the bathroom's doorknob. I cycled more slowly, and much less. One afternoon, several weeks later, I was late for my train, and ran for it, jumping through the fast diminishing space between the closing doors with a familiar sense of satisfaction. Once I was seated, book already out and open at the bookmark, my chest burned and my arms and legs tingled with a pins-and-needles sensation so aggressive it bordered on violence. I almost but not quite had to stop reading. Two hours later, interviewing a band whose new album I liked very much, I still hadn't quite got my breath back. 'You okay?' said the singer.

This, I finally acknowledged to myself, was disconcerting.

A week later, a concert with a friend. My friend is unnecessarily tall; I am significantly shorter. As we made our way from the Tube to the venue, I struggled to keep up with his Monty Python silly walk, and called out for him to slow down. We laughed about it, but even as I did so, I knew that it wasn't funny. Over a bite to eat afterwards, I found I could not drink my wine. A single swallow caused a muffled implosion inside my skull, and an abrupt sensation of tilting nausea. In its stead I ordered something called a Passionfruit & Orange Cooler. It came served with a straw. Again we laughed.

I had a whole week of normality after that, everything reasserting itself. Relief. I rescued my trunks from the bathroom doorknob, wrapped them in a towel, and jumped on my bike. A day later, fever, shakes and wretchedness.

Elena suggested I visit the doctor.

It was a joke in our house, perpetuated by myself alone, that our doctor would have made a good Nazi commandant. It was the severity of her manner, her thin-lipped impatience, that made her patients, like me, quake, and which turned any complaint into nothing more than yet another hypochondriac episode. 'And do close the door on your way out.'

I went anyway. She did not look up from the keyboard as she typed. While she did so, I talked. I recounted my symptoms, making light of them. Was I, she wondered, going through any stress at the moment? Some kind of emotional fallout? Everything all right at home? My answers caused her to sigh, and to suggest a blood test. I left, and closed the door behind me.

The results, a week later, came back negative. I was fine, panic over. Trouble was, I wasn't. Cycling was now all uphill, in the strictly metaphorical sense. I could no longer manage the three miles to my younger daughter's nursery without feeling like I was about to collapse. After my final attempt at swimming – though slowly now, and patiently, with no pretence of speed – I cancelled my gym membership, belatedly convinced I needed an extended period of recuperation. But from what? I half-heartedly hoped that the gym, keen for my monthly payments to resume, would try to tempt me back with special offers, new incentives, one month free. But there was nothing. I was immediately forgotten.

There was now not a week that went by without my feeling utterly dreadful in some new way. I was no expert in the field of flu, or its associated symptoms, but I had come to know it intimately, its tell-tale signs perpetually gathering in my sinuses, the backs of my eyes, my muscles. I would become sluggish, a deep ache in my legs, and in the parts of the spine that only an osteopath would be able to correctly identify. I found myself in bed by 10 most nights, often put there by my kindly, concerned wife before she went back downstairs to an adult existence, a book, a little TV, Mumsnet on the iPad.

Time passed, but my misery didn't. Perhaps I was now merely one of the 10 per cent of Britons who suffer from TATT, Tired All the Time, a vague sort of syndrome and evident epidemic that affects 10 million of us. Was that it? I made another appointment with the GP, a locum this time, and friendlier. She asked the same questions, and suggested more blood tests, different ones. 'Let's make an appointment again in, say, two weeks. Meantime, take it easy. Rest.'

The blood test was the fasting kind. No food after six o'clock the evening before. My appointment was for 9.30 a.m. I awoke in the morning with the girls, shortly before seven. I was starving. The usual whirlwind of getting two small children cleaned, dressed, fed and out the door kept me occupied, and I arrived at the surgery with 20 minutes to spare. My rumbling stomach howled out to everyone in the waiting room for attention.

I was called in after 10. 'Busy morning,' said the nurse as she tied a rubber flex around my arm. I watched the veins in my forearm rise, thought of Renton in *Trainspotting*, and turned to look the other way, testing my eyesight out on the chart pinned to the door: Z H S C T F X U.

She took a lot of blood, enough to fill six small test tubes. I asked what they were testing for, and she did respond, but it went in one ear and out the other before I could commit any of her answers to memory.

'All done,' she said, smiling.

I rolled down my sleeve, smiled back, and stood. The ceiling tilted promptly towards me. I hadn't expected it to.

'Oh. You're looking terribly pale,' the nurse said from somewhere in my peripheral vision. 'Do you want to lie down for a bit?'

I laughed, offered up the inevitable blush, and told her I would be fine. I pulled my coat on, said goodbye, then walked up the sloping corridor as it telescoped before me in a way I might have enjoyed had I the faculties, right then, to do so. I needed to sit down, and quickly. The reception area was full. I saw lots of bodies, but all the faces were blurred. There were no spare seats. My back, I realised, was soaking.

I stumbled through reception on leaden feet. A love song came on the radio, one I hadn't heard in years. As I reached the front door, it swung open, and in walked a boy, possibly 16, 17. His out-of-focus face was the last thing I saw. Beneath me, my legs had stopped working. I was pitching forward now, cleaving the air, and was not raising my arms to break my fall, even though the raising of arms to break a fall is an instinctive action. My head smashed onto the side of the door, and everything went black.

I imagine at this point there must have been raised voices, shouting, perhaps a cry for help. I have a low embarrassment threshold, the slightest public faux pas enough to make me rigid with anxiety, so I'm glad I heard none of it. But gradually I became aware of people on either side of me, and movement. Hands were tucked up under my armpits, and I was being dragged forwards. 'Can you walk?' somebody, female, asked me. A ludicrous question. Of course I could walk.

I couldn't walk. My legs were rubber.

'Deary me,' said a voice, the commandant's.

Now I was in the doctor's room, laid out cadaverously on a long white table. The table had joints, and could tilt up and down as required, and now I was being tilted backwards, my head hanging towards the floor. 'Let's get your blood circulating again,' said the nurse. 'You gave us quite a fright there, you know.'

'Fetch him some tea,' ordered the doctor. 'Plenty of sugar.'

'I'd prefer coffee,' I managed.

Elena was on a promise. Her mother, widowed for five years but reborn as a result and full of adventure, wanted to see New York. She, Elena and Elena's cousin were going for a full week. It was June, the perfect time to see the city.

'You'll be fine, yes?'

I gave the answer that was expected, that I wanted to give, but by now I had been unwell for six months. I had adapted accordingly, and in this way found that I could manage, more or less. Life had shrunk. In many ways, the recession the country was going through had played to my favour: there was no money to send journalists all over the world any more, and so instead we were being reintroduced to the marvels of the telephone, and its 21st-century upgrade, Skype. Now I could to all intents and purposes meet people from every country on earth while never leaving my room, and never changing out of my sweatpants.

I missed the perpetual thrill of being somewhere else, but I did not miss the jet lag, nor US customs, and besides, I was not yet being denied work. There was always an endless stream of visitors to London, and so I could meet people here instead. If there was less work, that had nothing to do with my being unwell; things were changing, everybody was having to make do.

Several times a week, then, I would take public transport into town for work appointments, now resisting the temptation to cycle everywhere but instead restricting my movements accordingly, and conserving what, it was now clear, were my fast-diminishing reserves of energy. I would arrive home tired, but fine. I began to rest more, to take things slower. It enabled me to cope, and I needed to cope. My swimming trunks had been put away, at the bottom of a drawer, and with them any semblance of a daily fitness regime I may have had. No more would my wife compliment me on my swimmer's shoulders, but then she had only ever done that once, and even then it wasn't really a compliment, merely an observation. Beneath my sweatpants, meanwhile, my calf muscles were growing softer. If I cycled at all now, it was for no more than a few minutes, either to the school to pick up my eldest daughter, or to the train, for which I no longer ran; if one was already on the platform as the station came into my view, I would resolve to miss it. How hard could it be, really, to wait 15 minutes until the next one?

Weekends had become quiet, spent here, at home and in the neighbourhood, where there were more than enough shops, if shops were what we craved. Everything else could wait.

That last round of blood tests, all six test tubes' worth, had come back negative. On paper, I was an advert for radiant health. The doctor, by now frustrated by her inability to offer a clinical diagnosis, referred me to an immunologist. I did not know what an immunologist was, but it put me in mind of tropical diseases. What would an immunologist want with me? A letter came from the hospital in due course, informing me that my appointment was three months away. It was scheduled for the third week of June. Elena went to New York in the second week of that month. For six days, I would be a single parent, which in my current status would prove a challenge. But then I have always liked a challenge.

Something unexpected happens within the family dynamic when one parent is out of the picture. When there is only one of you, the children can no longer play one off the other, and so the fireworks that can so frequently detonate remain largely dormant. In its place is a most pleasant, if surely temporary, synergy.

The six days we spent together were lovely. We all missed Elena, but we spoke to her regularly on the phone, and the photographs she emailed back suggested they were having fun. Amaya and Evie, then five and three, ate dinner every night without complaint, and fell asleep after the bedtime story far quicker than I had been anticipating. Even the arguments they had fizzled out quickly. I enjoyed their company, and looking in on them last thing at night, fast asleep, mouths open, limbs akimbo, I felt the fiercest, most prideful love for both.

But the physical requirements took a lot out of me, those perfunctory day-to-day trials that face any parent: taking one child to school by bike, and then another, by bus, to the crèche, the journey invariably delayed because three-year-olds dawdle, stop and sniff on route like dogs do, the round-trip taking an hour and a half. Then repeated at 3.20, arriving home in time for a dinner that needed, quickly, to be cooked.

They were in bed by 7.45 and, if I was lucky, asleep by nine. By nine, I was catatonic, my limbs unaccountably heavy. I laughed this off, embarrassed by it. Parents, single parents, do this all the time; my own mother did. Tiredness was nothing to be overly concerned about. It's what sleep was designed to help alleviate. And each night I would sleep very soundly indeed. But I would wake each morning desperate to sleep more.

At the weekend, there were parties to take the girls to, and presents to buy for both to take with them. By the end of Sunday, an eventful day that comprised broken crockery, an argument with a train driver, tears and laughter, I sat on the sofa alone, the girls asleep upstairs, and attempted to tune in properly to what my body was trying to tell me. I did not yet recognise its new language, but was aware at least of a cacophony. It is not enough to say that I felt tired. It was more than that, deeper, more profound, quite terrifying. I barely had the strength to reach for the remote control. My bed, a flight of stairs up, was unthinkable.

Elena called from JFK before boarding her flight.

'I know I'm always complaining about being tired,' I told her, 'but this is different. It's . . . *more*.'

She would be home shortly after dawn. I was glad. I needed her.

A week later, we visited friends in Wales. I didn't much want to go, but it had been scheduled. Wales was hilly. Physical exercise would be required.

On the Saturday, after lunch, we walked down one very steep incline, past fields dotted with sheep and horses and assorted Welsh people. The girls complained all the way. Their legs hurt; they were tired. You've seen one sheep, you've seen them all. Our friend suggested he walk back up to the house alone and fetch the car to bring us back. I rolled my eyes and tutted. Kids, eh? We both laughed. But once he had gone, I crouched down and hugged them both in gratitude. I wouldn't have been able to make it back up the hill either.

A few days later, I would see the immunologist. I was looking forward to it. He would be able to pinpoint what was wrong with me, and tell me how to get better. I'd had enough of this ongoing exhaustion, the nagging sense of a forever-encroaching flu. It got in the way of everything, it was boring, tiresome and dull. But tomorrow I would have a plan, a diagnosis, a course of antibiotics perhaps, magic pills, light at the end of the tunnel.

What I didn't know, what I *couldn't* know, was that by 10 o'clock tomorrow morning, everything would change and, somewhat melodramatically, life would never be the same again.

Two

My appointment with the immunologist is for 10 o'clock. I will have dropped Amaya off at school by 8.55, and the hospital is barely a 10-minute ride away. Under normal circumstances, I would have cycled home first, done a bit of work, and perhaps played a quick tournament of 8 Ball Pool on the iPad — *two* tournaments if I didn't win the first — then left at 9.50. But under normal circumstances, I wouldn't have been seeing an immunologist at all.

And so I decide to cycle slowly straight from school, a journey that takes me through a cemetery and up an unavoidable hill. I try to ignore the fierce asthmatic burn in my chest and the tremble in my legs as I lock my bike and orient myself.

Inside the hospital, the corridors lead to more corridors, which lead to a lift, a crowded reception area and a waiting room whose walls are the colour of oatmeal. While I wait, I wonder whether I should be nervous. I am in a place full of sick people, after all. Down yet another corridor, there is a series of doors into which people disappear when they are summoned; I do not know which of them are going in to see my doctor, whom I shall call here Dr Dolittle, if only because for me that was what he did do: little. From the looks on the faces of some of them afterwards, I realise that they go in as people and re-emerge as patients, their eyes downcast, a look of either grim determination or bewildered shock on their faces. I close my book and wait anxiously.

Eventually, my name is called, reliably mispronounced. Dr Dolittle is tall and pleasant-seeming. Like the doctors on television, he wears a white coat. It flaps around his grey trousers as he moves swiftly from the door to his chair. His office is small and narrow, more oatmeal on the walls, a window that looks out onto nothing much of anything. He tells me to sit and, multi-tasking already, suggests I tell him what is wrong while he reads through the notes sent to him by the GP. He nods a lot, and makes an agreeable sound from the back of his throat that I find soothing. He asks if I have undergone any emotional fall-out. A death in the family? How is my marriage? He asks what I do for a living, and looks up when I tell him. He asks how one goes about getting a book published – he has an idea for one – and so for a while we talk about this instead.

Then we get back to the subject at hand. To illustrate the limitations of my mysterious condition, I tell him what I did yesterday, that I had four jobs, all in town, with ample time to get from one appointment to the next. But because I haven't been feeling very well of late, I did not rush from one to the next, and did not take unnecessary diversions. I didn't hire a Boris bike and cycle over Tower Bridge for the sake of it, or phone a friend to meet them across town for a quick sandwich. Instead, I sat in cafés alone, pacing myself, conserving energy. I tell him that my condition has required me to take things slower, and that I tire easily. These are not pleasant sensations, and it doesn't suit me, but I have almost learned how to operate, and exist, at this temporarily slower pace.

This prompts more noises from the back of his throat. A good sign, I decide.

'I must say,' he says, apropos, as far as I can tell, of nothing, 'you don't strike me as particularly depressed.'

'No,' I agree.

'Because that's what we normally look for in situations like this, where the condition might be chronic fatigue.'

The two words fall with a thunk at my feet, like a dropped bag of potatoes. *Chronic fatigue*. Which means what, exactly? Very very very tired? This is the first time anyone has suggested this, with specific reference to *me*. Instinctively, I shirk from it. It is a label that won't stick. It has nothing to do with me.

'Or ME, as it's sometimes also known, although the two are quite different.'

He asks if I sleep well, whether I am good at relaxing.

I have heard of ME, or myalgic encephalomyelitis, before, of course. It's a relic from the '80s, yuppie flu. All in the mind. It doesn't exist, not really. Not a medical condition, per se. Afflicts the highly driven, the rapaciously ambitious, those who still believe that greed is good.

He asks if I have ever considered yoga. And then he says: 'Could you afford to stop working and live on your wife's wages for a year?'

I look up at him now, confused at what he has just said, and at what I think my ears have just heard. He is still taking notes, pursing his lips, and smiling, perhaps to himself.

'No,' I reply. 'Why? Do I need to?'

He laughs. It had been a joke, just a joke. I didn't get it. 'No, no,' he says. 'Just a worst-case scenario, that's all.'

More notes now, eyes cast down on the page, and he says to me that in his experience such conditions are usually linked to emotional issues. He reiterates that I don't appear to show any signs of depression, so maybe it is something else, but my symptoms are nevertheless consistent with some form of fatigue. And if fatigue persists for more than six months, and mine has, then it is given the awful appellation *chronic*.

I have been with him for 10 minutes now; I see him glance at the clock. Turning to me, he offers his diagnosis. I have post-viral fatigue. The virus – flu, presumably – has been in my body for many months now, I have proved incapable of successfully fighting it, and as a result it has worn me comprehensively down. My body needs rest until it can be fully free from the virus. There is no definitive way of telling when this might be. He says that it is important for me to walk at least half an hour every day. Graded exercise therapy, he calls it. And if I can't do half an hour, then do at least 15 minutes. 'This,' he stresses, 'is important.'

Sitting in my chair by his desk, I feel six years old again. I am confused. Why wouldn't I be able to walk for half an hour a day? I have just told him that I had been out for hours yesterday. I want to tell him this, remind him, ask him to explain more, but my time is up. He stands, chuckling good-naturedly, and leads me to the door.

'You'll be fine,' Dr Dolittle says, a paternal hand on my shoulder. 'You'll be fine. But do some yoga! And relax!'

He gives me a sheet of paper advertising CBT classes at another hospital for sufferers of ME and chronic fatigue syndrome (CFS), waves me goodbye, then ushers in his next patient, a young woman who doesn't make eye contact with me as our paths cross.

I cycle home, downhill all the way. It's a busy day, two deadlines outstanding, but before starting work, I google those threatening acronyms, ME and CFS. 'Significantly debilitating' are the first two words that stand out from the screen to catch my eye. Bad Google; I had been hoping, inexplicably, for a little moderation in its explanation, not shock tactics. 'No known cure', I read, by which time my eyesight is failing me, lightbulb flashes exploding in my retinas. I read on. Because everything we experience now must be filtered through the world of celebrity, I find myself scrolling through a long list of famous people who have had it: rock stars and film stars, writers, actors. One describes it as 'a living hell'. Another has not been able to leave her bedroom for over three years. Another still requires the use of a wheelchair. I am skimming now, unable to take in a sentence to its full stop, palpably terrified of what I might read next. More than a million Americans have it, 600,000 Brits and rising. The 'total annual cost burden' to the USA is around $24 billion. I see endless entries that feature the word 'controversy'. This is an illness, a condition, that seems to make a lot of people angry, reactionary, even murderous in intent.

By the time I find another reference to it having no known cure, my right hand is grappling for the mouse and clicking away. I will not be googling this again. I put it out of my mind. There is work to be done, lunch, the school run, a resumption of my normal life.

My area of journalism, the most ephemeral and throwaway, rarely takes me anywhere officious and grown up, and so I am surprised to find myself, two days later, in an hour-long queue to get into the Houses of Parliament. The queue itself is nothing compared with Heathrow's Terminal 3, but the security measures here are even more thorough. We are all potential security threats, insurrectionists, shoe bombers, likely wielders of belt buckles, and so studiously methodical pat-downs are mandatory, and terribly time-consuming. It is convincingly warm enough today to suggest that summer has arrived. I am overdressed in the only thing my wardrobe offered up as notionally smart: a pair of newish jeans, a shirt and a pair of shoes I last wore to somebody's wedding.

The queue is not moving. I am accustomed to queues, but my legs are beginning to ache. It is a powerful ache. The more I become aware of it, the worse it gets, and I fight a growing impulse to leave, to find a seat, to sit down and let whatever it is that is happening to me pass.

By the time I reach the metal detectors, I am swamped in relief. They can have my shoes, my belt, my bag. I don't care any more. The security staff, at least, are a good-natured bunch, smiling where their airport counterparts can only frown, and at last I am within the House itself. I make a beeline for the café, where I buy nothing, just sit and take the weight off my feet. Disarmingly, I am huffing and puffing, and hot under the collar in a way that has nothing to do with the heat.

I walk through the House's grand hall, which hums with activity. The BBC's Nick Robinson is in one alcove, doing a piece to camera; somebody from ITV is doing a similar thing in the alcove opposite. MPs recognisable from TV and lurid sex-life exposés walk leisurely past, hands in pockets, trailed by minions in their wake. Instinctively, I look out for *The Thick of It's* Malcolm Tucker. I am here to attend a speech on smoking that will condemn the government's continued public ban on nicotine. Presumably because the subject matter is a controversial one, the venue for the speech has been banished to the very end of the building, down several long corridors and out into a room that flanks the Thames which, this close up, looks sad and brown and full of sickness. Everybody here is out on the terrace, smoking copiously (cigarettes, pipes, cigars), many carelessly tossing their butts into the water afterwards.

The artist David Hockney, one of the guest speakers, arrives and people gather excitedly around him. A drink is bought for him at the busy bar, and the bar remains busy because the speeches are delayed. I look around, but find nowhere to sit, and I need, gravely, to do just that. I lean against the low wall outside and stare into a river too brown to offer back my reflection. I wonder what is happening to me, my legs. At the rim of my consciousness is an increasing awareness of a ballooning fear.

A torturous hour later – I leave early – the Circle Line takes me to Victoria, and from here I go overland to Clapham Junction and change for the train home. It is rush hour, and my carriage is packed. I have to stand. By now the urgency to sit is almost suffocating. I close my eyes and reach out for a handrail, willing the journey to pass quickly. I remember that my bike is waiting for me at the train station, and feel both relief that I don't have to walk home and frantic at the prospect of having to cycle.

I make it back and go straight up to bed. Elena, still cooking dinner for the children, comes up. 'You all right?' The girls follow behind, jumping on the bed, using my chest as a pommel horse. They laugh and shout, and both talk over the other to tell me about their day. Drawn by the smell of cooking, they one by one go back downstairs again, and I roll over, turn on the radio, but hear nothing. My head is all over the place, thoughts racing.

Something is happening, I realise, something bad. A careless comment from a medic lacking in people skills sent me online, where I found at last concrete proof that what has been wrong with me these past six months is in fact serious, and is likely to get worse. *No known cure.* When Woody Allen is in the grip of a hypochondriac episode in *Hannah and her Sisters*, it is funny. He plays it for laughs, considering the slightest headache a tumour about to happen, then casts blindly about to find a religion quick, a willing God to accept him before it's too late. I had not been much of a hypochondriac before. Am I one now?

The following day, I interview a 39-year-old schoolteacher who, six months previously, became aware that he was developing a limp in his right foot. I had originally planned to travel to Somerset to meet him at his house, but the exhaustion I had felt in Parliament has yet to lift; we speak on the telephone instead. He tells me that he had noticed it, the limp, when he went up the stairs at school. 'It kind of flopped.' He found the cycle into work harder each morning, and then noticed that he had lost a lot of weight from his right thigh. His GP agreed that this was 'sinister' and he was referred for tests. 'Before he sent me away, he made me promise not to go onto Google,' he tells me. A month later came the diagnosis: motor neurone disease. 'It was absolutely devastating.'

I do not know what to say to him. This poor man, who would go on to campaign for greater funding into understanding and treatment for MND, refused to let his indomitable spirit dampen, at least for as long as he was capable. He is hopeful, he says, in the face of no hope at all. 'I've my wife to think about, my children.' I admire him for his bravery, and in his see that I have none. His experience casts mine into shadow, his being major, mine comparatively minor. But there are parallels: one day he was fine, the next day he was not. His would, and did just two cruel years later, come to an abrupt conclusion; mine, with its *no known cure* boast, might also prove a life sentence.

The panic attack, when it comes, is a new experience. I have never had one before. It is not quite as dramatic as I might have expected. I require no brown paper bag in which to breathe, and I do not scream, or flail, or pull at hair strands. But it is a panic attack; the internet confirms it.

'A panic attack', says the NHS web page dealing with stress, anxiety and depression, 'is a rush of intense psychological and physical symptoms. They can be frightening and happen suddenly, often for no clear reason. They usually last between five and 20 minutes, and although it may feel as though you are in serious trouble, they aren't dangerous and shouldn't cause any physical harm. You may feel an overwhelming sense of fear and a sense of unreality, as if you are detached from the world around you. You may experience physical symptoms such as: palpitations, sweating, trembling, shortness of breath, chest pain.'

The paragraph is illustrated with a photograph. In the middle of what looks like a pink jelly mould is a red button upon which the word PANIC is written. You sense, looking at this picture, that if you touched it, it would wobble.

It is a Saturday afternoon, and hot. Wimbledon is into its second week. The girls, cooped up in the house all morning, are ready for air, to open the front door and run in any direction their feet take them. I have been unusually quiet all morning, Elena tells me. I have had much to think on. I have so many questions, and no idea to whom I can pose them.

Several years later, I will speak to an NHS chronic fatigue specialist, Professor Peter White, who will ask me why I didn't seek a second opinion if Dolittle's was so unsatisfying. At first I won't know how to answer this question. My truthful response would be that I didn't think to, that I thought the only people who asked for second opinions were those in films, or Americans. Perhaps second opinions were requested when people didn't trust the original doctor's prognosis. I had little reason to distrust Dr Dolittle; I just wished he had explained things a little more to me.

'Ah, well, the NHS is not what it was, I'm afraid,' Professor White will say. 'Twenty years ago, you would have had an hour's consultation, at least. But we are facing cuts of around £150,000 a year. We have more referrals, less money, fewer resources.'

He will say that four out of 10 cases of CFS are misdiagnosed by doctors and immunologists, 'and so if you are not given the right diagnosis, it's no surprise when the treatment they offer doesn't work.'

But, as I say, that would not be until several years later.

Meanwhile, Dolittle's diagnosis was that I had some kind of post-viral fatigue, but the treatment he recommended was for CFS and ME. In the absence of my wherewithal to demand a second opinion, I don't know what to do. I need information, advice, but not of the hysterical, online kind. Dr Dolittle did say I should contact him again if I wanted to attend one of his classes, but at the moment I do not feel best disposed towards him. I cannot say that I particularly want to see the man again. Besides, Elena googled him. A number of people seem to have been upset by him; he is the subject of several blogs, their complaints all the more powerful because they are so competently written. A colleague of Elena's at work, also recently diagnosed with a post-viral condition, wrote a letter of complaint to the hospital after a consultation with him.

I still need help, however. But from where?

Closing the door to the kitchen and my family, I sit in a chair in the living room and stare out of the window. A concrete block is pushing on my ribcage. I am having difficulty breathing.

Elena comes in. She looks at me with such compassion and worry that tears spring to my eyes. And then, abruptly, I start to cry. Behind her, the girls bound in, laughing and shouting. They stop short. They look at me in incomprehension. They have not seen me cry before.

'I'll take them out,' Elena says, and ushers them back into the kitchen.

Before she leaves, she gives me a Post-it note on which is written a number and the words: ME/CFS Helpline. While I slept last night, she went online looking for help.

'Call them,' she says. 'Call them, and see what they say. And then call me, yes?'

I watch them leave the house, walk down the garden path and away. Then I go upstairs to my room in order to watch them from the window as they round the corner before crossing the main road. My girls, in summer dresses and hats, are on their scooters, Elena walking proudly behind them. I become tearful again.

I attempt to calm myself down. I have to behave rationally, coolly. If I am ill, and if I am about to get worse, then there are things I need to do, now, quickly, just in case. I have one deadline outstanding. I was planning to write it up on Monday, but I write it up now, on Saturday, while I still can. I have no idea what state I might be in on Monday.

It is not a big piece; it takes me an hour. It's only when I finish it that the panic returns. I find the Post-it note and dial the number. It starts ringing, but abruptly I hang up. I almost laugh at the teenage anticipation that runs through me, the prospect of having someone answer my call making me nervous and tongue-tied. I dial again, then hang up again upon the realisation that I have no idea what to say, or the order in which to say it. And so I make some notes.

I rehearse out loud what it is I want to say, the questions I might ask, and then call. The number rings and rings. I check the website, which says that it is open 24 hours a day, 365 days a year. I try again, then again. No answer.

I decide to watch the tennis, but cannot concentrate. The weight on my chest intensifies. I look out of the window and watch people pass, heading into town. I would feel sorry for myself, but I'm too busy feeling scared. The urge to cry is powerful. I'm having trouble breathing. What is happening to me? I think I'm having palpitations. I've become that pink jelly mould, PANIC in capital letters.

I call the helpline again, and the helpline's failure to pick up seems only to confirm that I am in an awful lot of trouble here.

The girls arrive home. Elena arranges the children in front of the television with a snack while she and I retreat into the kitchen, closing the door behind us for the first of what will become a depressingly regular tête-à-tête. She reveals herself as good in a crisis, steady and reassuring. I am glad I married her.

The helpline people continue to not pick up, but NHS Direct does. The lady at the end of the line listens patiently, then arranges an emergency appointment for me within the hour, just after a dinner I have no appetite for. The doctor on call, a young

Indian man on crutches ('Rugby injury,' he tells me, beaming) is kind and full of empathy. He shakes his head and clutches at it comically when I relay the immunologist's diagnosis, and tells me he is sick of doctors who forget that their patients are not just cases but real people, and often vulnerable ones. He tells me nothing Elena hasn't already told me, but it's nice to hear soothing words from someone with a stethoscope around his neck. He tells me I've had a shock, that I'm dealing with a shock, and I'll be fine. As for dealing with whatever this post-viral fatigue may be, he doesn't quite know what to say. Perhaps I could go back to my GP and ask for their help?

Back at home, I go to bed early, and wake early on Sunday morning. For the first few seconds, my mind is blank. Then I remember. Everything is different now. I shall have to get used to it.

Chronic fatigue is an umbrella term for a variety of conditions with overlapping symptoms. Fatigue is the one constant, but it can manifest itself in all sorts of ways, including depression, muscle pain, constant headaches. There is a distinct difference between ME and CFS, but when Professor White, one of the world's leading experts on the subject, explains them to me several years later, they sail far above my head, borne aloft by the buoyancy of complicated medical terms with far too many syllables to them. ME, it seems, is the more serious strand, which I suppose means CFS is its more manageable sibling.

Either way, neither has a particular pathology present. There is no blood test to confirm them. This is why GPs are so quick to refer patients elsewhere: they cannot diagnose it with the same emphasis they can with, say, lung cancer or heart disease. Those are concrete conditions; this one is an irritating enigma.

'If it looks like CFS and smells like CFS,' Professor White will say, 'it could very likely be something else. It could be anaemia, sleep disorder, depression. But, still, CFS is the likely diagnosis to reach for.'

Consequently, more than half a million people in Britain currently labour under the impression they have it when they don't (and I am one of them, though I won't learn this key piece of information for another three years, when I see a new consultant), while many hundreds, possibly thousands, are still awaiting confirmation. If you have had persistent symptoms of fatigue for more than six months, and if no other medical explanation for those symptoms is forthcoming, then you are duly diagnosed. A course of treatment is then recommended, but recommendations differ wildly. The NHS favours Dr Dolittle's graded exercise therapy (GET), as well as mindfulness cognitive behavioural therapy. Alternative practitioners, of which, as I will discover, there are a great many, tend to disagree with the NHS, and not merely on knee-jerk principle. GET, they say, is in fact dangerous, and will only make the patient worse, even set back their recovery. And of those who have attempted GET and suffered, a select but belligerent few have taken to sending their doctors death threats. They don't carry the threats out, but it does get them column inches in newspapers, which in turn gives them a dubious reputation. It is for this reason that, before he would agree to be interviewed by me, I had to convince Peter White that I wasn't another death-threatening crackpot (my terminology, not his) out for his blood.

I first come across Professor Peter White in the media. On 5 May 2013, the cover of the *Sunday Times* magazine is made up to look like a blackmail letter, words cut out and stuck unevenly, and thus sinisterly, together. It reads: **YOU EVIL BAStARDS . . . WE'RE gOING to CUT YOUR balls off. STay out of ThIS . . . time is running OUT for you ALL. PRAY TO gOD for FORgiveness.**

Underneath, it continues: 'Scientists Under Siege. Doctors are facing death threats simply for suggesting ME, the chronic fatigue illness, is all in the mind.'

I do not read this article when it first appears. I am still too raw and vulnerable, and the idea of being so closely associated with murderous loons does not appeal, so I file the magazine away for another, indeterminate time.

Eventually, a year later, I get around to it. It is bewildering stuff, focusing on a hardcore element of purported sufferers – no more than 50 to 80 nationwide, by all accounts, and *purported* because the article asserted that some were believed not to have any condition at all but merely an inexplicable axe to grind – motivated to commit hate campaigns because the field of science had deemed ME a psychological problem rather than one caused by a virus. These 50 to 80, and quite possibly many thousands besides, believe instead that it is viral, that you catch it via glandular fever or a persistent flu. They are convinced it is similar to HIV ('the hidden AIDS', they call it). It is spread by infection.

From what I have come to understand of the condition, this seems unlikely, but a medical paper from 2009 was cited suggesting that a retrovirus called XMRV had been identified in more than two thirds of ME patients tested. Proof? Actually, no. The paper's findings were subsequently deemed unreliable, impossible to substantiate, but this seemed not to matter to the hardcore, or else was easy to ignore, and so they raged on. The core gripe is this: we are being overlooked by the NHS. The condition is not being given its due attention, much less sufficient funding. How, then, can we find a cure without the necessary funding?

And so they are angry. And even though many of their lives are blighted by the physical and mental exhaustion typical of the condition, they do manage to summon up rather impressive reserves of energy necessary to wage really quite sinister campaigns of the kind more normally associated with radical anti-abortionists in Bible Belt America.

Several prominent UK doctors received death threats; one had had a panic button installed in his house as a precaution. The *Sunday Times* article was unable to quote any of the hardcore because the hardcore don't have much faith in a sympathetic ear from the mainstream press. It did quote one campaigner, though, a former vet convinced he had caught ME 'through having sex with his girlfriend in the early 1990s. He was struck off by the British Veterinary Association after inadvertently killing a cat, and was convicted of indecent assault on a 12-year-old girl in 2004 – both incidents precipitated, he says, by a combination of ME and the heavy drinking he fell into in an effort to self-medicate.'

I find I have to read this paragraph twice, just in case I misread it the first time around. I hadn't.

The article suggests that 600,000 people in the UK currently suffer from ME. Fifty to 80 radicals, then, is a tiny proportion of that, and so hardly representative. You can find crackpots anywhere. Nevertheless, and largely due to articles like this, sufferers tend to be tarred with the same brush: we are crackpots, all.

There is no single agreed-upon way of treating the condition. Different experts come at it differently; it is up to us to sift through them all and decide, for ignorant reasons or enlightened ones, which suits us best. This can take years and cost a great deal of money.

Some specialists look to early childhood trauma as a potential root of the problem. Others do not. Some say you must rest, listen to your body, ingest as many vitamins as possible, do yoga, meditate. Others say you have to fight back, regain control over your mind, and your body will follow. It is a mental disorder; a purely physical one. You can infect others with it, can catch it from unprotected sex.

Amid these competing voices, there appears to be at least some concrete evidence: 'Your personal history does play a significant role to later abnormal stress responses,' Professor White will say to me when I meet him. 'If you have had a childhood adversity of some kind, then it changes your stress responses as an adult.'

In other words, it is the way we cope after having fallen ill that determines the path of our recovery.

'We now know the epigenetic response,' he'll say. 'Childhood trauma doesn't change your DNA, but it does change the expression of your genes, particularly those that determine your stress response, and particularly your cortisol response.'

Cortisol is our main stress hormone, and people with CFS have 40 per cent less cortisol than those without.

'This means that your adrenal axis is low, which means that when you have to deal with the added stress – a persistent case of adrenalin, say – then you do not always cope quite as well.'

Fatigue, then, is merely one of many paths we can go down when we burn out. It remains chronic if we stress over the illness unduly, because the more we stress, the longer we will stay ill, and the longer we are ill, the more we stress. In many cases, it is difficult not to. Burnout is increasingly common these days, in some cases unavoidable. A great many of us will eventually burn out in one way or another. There are many manifestations to it: heart attack, stroke, aneurysm. There is a suggestion that certain cancers are the result of excessive, prolonged stress. In most cases, the way back is slow, and requires methodical planning, and occasionally a complete overhaul of one's lifestyle. Some people find God, or spirituality. Some make a full recovery, others don't. Those who do can be accused by those who don't of never having had CFS in the first place. Long-time sufferers, at least those portrayed in the media, can be bitter – but then who wouldn't be after years of illness?

However you choose to navigate it, it will be complicated, and will require very great levels of attention. Learning a foreign language would be easier, and quicker.

But which way to turn? There are so many competing voices. When your GP isn't on hand to offer a swift remedy, then you are forced to look elsewhere — specifically, into the world of alternative medicine — new waters for me. There is a proliferation of opinion here, and all manner of unlikely-sounding treatments are advocated. Some of the advice overlaps, plenty doesn't, and alternative practitioners tend to contradict one another vocally. The NHS can endorse none of them until concrete proof of a cure is offered. And there is no such proof yet.

For anyone newly initiated into the world of CFS (but still in denial), this can all be wildly disconcerting. I have not been properly ill before and, having been effectively dispensed with by the NHS, it seems I now have a choice on what to do and whom to follow. But I have no idea what I am doing, nor what I *should* be doing, no map, no single guide. It's bewildering.

And they say ignorance is bliss.

Three

Arranged on the kitchen table before me are pills, vitamins and a variety of purportedly energy-boosting supplements wielding serious names: Vegepa, D-Ribose, L-Glutathione, Acetyl L-Carnitine, Transdermal Magnesium. I have heard of none of these before, and when I look them up – and learn that one of them, the Glutathione, is an antioxidant preventing damage to important cellular components caused by reactive oxygen species such as free radicals and peroxides – I have little clearer idea of what good they might do. Vitamin D3 I have heard of, or think I have heard of, but not Coenzyme Q10, or Siberian ginseng, which by all accounts is preferable in this case to Korean ginseng, though I couldn't tell you why. There is also echinacea, selenium, chromium, vitamin C and niacinamide, and some BioCare multivitamins and minerals. They make for quite a haul, and lined up together they fill half the table.

It is breakfast time. The children file in and appraise the table quizzically.

'What are they for?' Evie asks.

It's a good question.

As my fatigue worsens, Elena has become my carer, spending hours on the internet during her lunch hour at work and each evening at home, trying to find a cure, a remedy, the best treatment. There is an awful lot of information online, inevitably too much, and it proves a muddy topic, endlessly argued over,

37

ridiculed and hotly contested, everybody with a strong opinion. It seems that any practitioner with a specialism in the field of fatigue is subject to criticism and official complaint. And so Elena has to read and reread, then cross-reference, and brace herself through the many hundreds of online comments from around the world while trying to maintain a cool head. All the proffered advice here has been both hailed for its effectiveness and derided for its quackery, the practitioners behind it either worshipped as gurus or scorned as charlatans. All of them are private and costly, their remedies time-consuming and not guaranteed. But then this is my new world now, and the path stretching out before me is riven with crazy paving.

The kitchen table with its pills and concoctions, then, is the result of Elena's findings to date, the advice that resonated most – namely, the recommendations of a certain general practitioner who, three years previously, had been struck off the NHS register after she continued to treat the condition outside of NHS guidelines. I question Elena's decision here, but she assures me that she has waded through all the hysteria prompted by the GP's sacking to learn that the doctor was quickly reinstated, and that from what she can see, the woman knows what she is talking about. Much of what Elena has read online has left her suspicious or else confused; this is one of the exceptions. According to this doctor, in the first flush of the condition, the body is still struggling against the virus. Before we can treat our own individual reaction to it, we have to get the body back to its optimal potential. It needs to recover and renew, and, Elena explains, these pills should help do just that. I am to take them daily, some on an empty stomach, others with meals, or after meals. Some look big enough to comprise a meal in themselves. Together, over time, it is suggested, their combination will restore within me all the energy the virus has depleted. I will feel their effects, and, with them, I will start to feel better.

It seems impossible I will ever be able to remember which to take when. Elena suggests a multi-pill dispenser that does the arranging for us. I refuse this on principle. A multi-pill dispenser brings with it the kind of connotations I don't want to consider just yet, of the elderly, the long-term ill. Instead, I get a felt-tip pen and write easy-to-read instructions on each, then arrange them on a cupboard shelf of their own, out of the children's reach.

Alongside the pills, it is also recommended I take something called transdermal magnesium, which the doctor has dubbed 'Magic Minerals'. Minerals are essential for the building of strong bones and teeth, for turning the food we eat into energy. Minerals can be found in meat, cereals, dairy products, vegetables, fruit and nuts. But right now I need an industrial amount, and so the 'Magic Minerals' come in an industrial-sized container. It looks like, and has the consistency of, sand. A heaped tablespoon, I read, is to be dissolved in tap water or juice, then swallowed. The label does draw attention to the fact that some people do not like the taste of the minerals. They can find this substance too unpleasant even to swallow. It is better for health reasons to swallow it, but if it proves too much for the sensitive palate, then there is always the transdermal option instead – spreading it on the skin, which will absorb it.

The whole thing is daunting, offering as it does concrete proof that I am really not very well at all. I need to make light of things, for myself and my audience: two intrigued children and my concerned wife. I mix an experimental glass, the powder making the water cloudy and thick. It is odourless. I offer it around. 'A health drink,' I call it. 'Like a smoothie, more or less.' Evie adopts a fierce expression, and pronounces: 'No.' Amaya allows the glass to touch her lips, then promptly retches, and passes the glass to her mother. Elena, always stoical, the calm in any storm, takes a gulp. What happens next is interesting. Her face folds in on itself as if lemon juice has just been squirted into her eyes. The bones in her neck become visible as her skin is pulled taut in a grimace. A strange noise emerges, possibly from the nostrils, and she fumbles to put the glass onto the nearest surface without spilling it. She sticks her tongue out and peels back her lips. The children look at her in horror. Once it is clear she isn't going to die, they laugh uncertainly. Then they all turn to look at me.

None of this bodes well. But I am determined to do whatever is deemed to be good, even if it is disgusting, and so I drink it. This is, after all, what the label suggests – the label written by a doctor who, I recall now, had initially been struck off for her unconventional methods, but no matter. Onwards. I drink, and I swallow. I react the way Elena did. The taste is almost beyond description: thick like olive oil, slick like petrol, and dauntingly strong, with an undertow of fungus. Every swallow prompts a gag, and a fatigue-defying dash to the toilet because surely I'm going to bring it up again.

'Maybe drink it slowly, in tiny sips, over the next few hours?' Elena gamely suggests.

For a full week, I do this. The glass sits threateningly on my desk, and every 15 minutes, I stop working to sip, gag, retch. But a week is all I can manage. One glass is enough to make me feel sick all day – it sits in my stomach like a tide that refuses to go out, and bubbles – and if seven days produces no discernible improvement in me, then it's too slow, and I've had enough.

By week two, I begin to ingest it transdermally. The experience offers little improvement. Its grainy, sand-like quality is not readily soluble, and so you don't so much smear it into the skin as scratch it in. Once applied, it forms an oily sheen which, the label suggests, should be allowed to settle for at least half an hour. I do it first thing in the morning, before my shower, then slip on an old T-shirt that soon becomes irreparably soiled, and make my way down to breakfast. I cannot lean back on the chair because the T-shirt is slick and sticky, and so I eat my toast sitting unnaturally upright. As it dries, it tightens and seems to pull everything upwards, like a cosmetic surgery procedure. If my belly button is below the waistband of my sweatpants before I apply it, then afterwards it's above.

'Your T-shirt is leaking,' Amaya tells me, a concerned look on her face.

After half an hour has passed, I can finally shower and rub the stuff off and into the drain. I repeat this process every day for months on end, and every day I think it best not to question too much what it is I am doing here, and to what end. I have had to put my critical faculties on hold, and content myself with the necessary fact that for the time being I must do precisely as I am told.

The fridge has been filling up, meanwhile, with red meat and broccoli. I have never been particularly fond of beef, finding it difficult to digest, and I would never eat it for lunch, but Elena insists I need the protein. The internet says so. So, no more quick sandwich in front of the TV, but rather a flash-fried sliver of bleeding cow, a fried egg and several stalks of green on the side.

Elena is now spending a lot of time on the computer, reading up on my condition. Of all the conditions to have, this is one of the less dramatic ones. There is little pizzazz to it, no fanfare, no ceremony. You are horribly, comprehensively tired, and that's it. It doesn't appear to be particularly progressive; it doesn't kill. There is no lump that needs excising, no radical treatment that, if successful, could do wonders for a doctor's success rate. Doubt over prognosis abounds, as does conflict over treatment. Despite the course of pills I am on, having been diagnosed by a registered NHS doctor, there is no course of pills recommended by the NHS.

If you can pinpoint why you might have developed it – if, that is, you are not one of the four in 10 to be misdiagnosed in the first place – then this might help with the subsequent treatment. Elena and I talk endlessly about this, wondering why this might have happened to me. What is its root? Why am I unable to answer the question the immunologist asked me, and the GP before him, relating to emotional fallout? Has there been any which I might have missed? Wouldn't I have been aware of it? Is it possible to be depressed without realising it?

Later, Professor Peter White will tell me that the majority of sufferers do not, in fact, suffer from depression at all, but before I meet with him, I am told that depression is often considered a key factor.

So I navel-gaze in an attempt to spot it lurking somewhere within me, aware that denial wields considerable power. I grew up with a mother prone to depression, though I always believed her depression to be more circumstantial than clinical. Either way, I got to know the signs, how it developed, how long a bout would last. I do not think I have ever had anything similar. I have all manner of daily anxieties, of course, but these to me are low- level, manageable, the everyday stuff of life, and certainly nothing that would result in something as powerful as this. Otherwise, everything is mostly fine, unspectacular, normal. If anything, I have always considered myself unaccountably lucky. I have been gifted with a wife and children whom I love very much. I have a job I respect and still covet, grateful to be able to live and breathe it. It has allowed me to see a lot of the world, and meet a lot of strange, fascinating people. I live in a nice enough house in a nice enough area, though naturally I would like a bigger house in a better area. I have a TV with a Live Pause function that never ceases to impress me. I sleep well. I wake happy. Don't I?

Things could of course be better, much. Life could be improved in any number of ways. How much time do you have?

I could be taller, stronger, fitter, with 20/20 vision. I could have more work, better pay, a regular salary like normal people, a turn of phrase like Clive James'. Editors would email me rather than waiting for me to email them, and would fight for the privilege of commissioning me. I could have been bequeathed, by some phantom aunt, a trust fund, buying me that most elusive of things: financial security. I could have more friends, *better* friends, the kind of children who liked what their father cooked for them, and who ate it without complaint. I wish I were more assertive, more confident, less timid.

And then there are the regrets. I wish I could have helped appease the rift between my mother and my grandmother before my mother died. I am still distraught, 30 years on, that I didn't follow 16-year-old Ruth Gibson up to her empty dormitory on our French school trip when I was 15, an invitation she would not make twice despite my pleading. I always wanted to travel on the Trans-Siberian Express, and haven't done yet. I regret letting certain friendships slide. I really shouldn't have bought those G-Star cargo trousers. I wish I'd run the London Marathon, just once.

Offer me a wish list that would make life better, and I will swiftly fill it. But mostly, I can't quite believe my luck. Or couldn't.

Try as I might, I cannot find any obvious contributing factors. And so perhaps my problem is less psychiatric and more fundamental, more basic. Perhaps, for whatever reason, I have simply been wired wrong, and don't possess the ability to cope with it all: with work, with parenthood, and with the endless pressures in the maintenance of both. I have somehow skewed my work-life balance irreparably, my DNA faulty, substandard. Everybody else can cope, but not me. I could, for a while, and I managed well enough, but then I crested over into middle age, and into less of a crisis than a full-on meltdown.

Is that it?

Did I ride too much, and for too long, on my adrenalin, always rushing, rarely resting, overlooking the importance of pacing, of relaxing, of quality of life? Hindsight tells me that my body clamoured for respite, a slower pace, for years, decades even, but I ignored it. My body needed one thing, my brain craved another, and so the former ultimately gathered together its disparate parts and downed tools in protest.

I should have been paying better attention. But I didn't. Does anyone?

I am paying attention now. I need to do something drastic, to acknowledge the diagnosis and to show – at least to myself – that I am belatedly taking it as seriously now as I should have then. And so immediately I stop chasing work with quite the same vigour I always have done.

Being able to do this is disconcertingly easy. The freelance life is rarely a particularly secure one, which is something I have always considered one of its more appealing traits: it keeps you keen. If you do not chase work, the work very rarely chases you. There are thousands of *me* out there, all with the same drive, the same 'YES!' mentality. Elena has often accused me of putting work before everything else. She is right. I was nearly late for my own wedding because of a last-minute deadline that interfered with me putting on my suit.

It is a bit late to suggest I have seen the error of my ways, not least as it was usually Elena who suffered due to my work, not me. But now I try, conspicuously and not a little self-consciously, to take things easy. After the girls have gone to school, and Elena to work, I linger on the sofa. But it feels wrong to be in front of the television, it feels lazy, so I read instead. The house is too quiet, and so I gravitate helplessly upstairs and switch on the computer. I cannot help it; it is where I am happiest, where I can relax.

I am currently writing a book for someone, a ghosting project. Though this qualifies for the term 'work', it is currently unpaid work. Nevertheless, it is intensive, and that suits me. I have been putting in eight-hour days on it for the past six months; at night I dream exclusively of re-writes. My plan now is to write merely for an hour, and then rest for an hour, and so on throughout the day.

Time flies when I work, the hours like minutes. Sat in front of the computer, writing to deadline, I feel like a car that has just been filled up with petrol, ready to go, a heavy foot on the accelerator. If I merely sit in a chair and stare at the wall instead, does this really qualify as proper relaxation? It doesn't settle my brain. Instead, my brain remains agitated, bored. It craves diversion, attention. The truth is I have no idea how to relax.

This needs to change. Humbled by my perpetual exhaustion, I begin to handle myself with exaggerated care. One afternoon after lunch – having quickly tired of all the red meat, I have now moved on to scrambled eggs and asparagus, protein and antioxidants – I stay rooted to the sofa and watch a film, but time drags. I can't go swimming, can no longer go out on my bike. I cannot even leave the house these days without it resulting in the most ravaging exhaustion, in which every muscle feels spent of all its energy, and I am flat as a punctured tyre, a good night's sleep doing precisely nothing to alleviate the symptoms.

This is hard to take in, and I struggle with it daily. I still have no real idea what is happening to me, nor why. I know that the vast array of vitamins I am taking each morning, the transdermal minerals included – total cost at well over £200 – appear to be doing nothing at all.

One day, feeling particularly down, I decide to write to Dr Dolittle, explaining the abrupt downward spiral that occurred after seeing him and telling him that I need answers, and that I would be very grateful if he could proffer some. It takes him over a month to respond.

He wrote that my reaction didn't surprise him, that it was not untypical of patients once they knew that something was seriously wrong. He suggested I ask my GP to refer me to my local hospital for some graded exercise therapy sessions.

In the meantime, I read a book, a memoir, about a writer's search for relief from the chronic pain he has been suffering for decades, and it is here, perhaps consciously for the first time, that I learn about the link between the mind and the body, and how *psychosomatic* – so often a term of ridicule, the suggestion that the illness is only ever 'in the mind' – has been accepted as fact in the East, specifically India, for centuries. Why wouldn't the mind influence the body, and vice versa? Why the shame in having a physical condition exacerbated by the mental response to it?

My life over the next few weeks shrinks in increments until it is wafer thin. No swimming, no cycling, no trips into town for work because I am not, for the time being, chasing work. I have one daily excursion, and it proves difficult enough: the school run. It's a 10-minute walk, so I cycle it in three. Because it is summer, we stop on the way home at the playground. We get back to the house perhaps an hour later, my body roaring its disapproval: prickles of extreme tiredness burning in my arms, my thighs, the backs of my eyes. My eyelids, I've become aware, ache, something I didn't know was possible. I crave only oblivion, to switch off to everything. If I could hibernate, I would.

Slowly, I start actively seeking journalism jobs again, *paying* jobs, sending emails to editors about jobs that, if commissioned, I can do on the phone or, via cab, in town. I do not tell them about my condition, of course, because they don't need to know. If the opportunity comes for a job overseas, I make excuses. I don't travel more than 10 miles for a job now. If nothing else, I am spared the jet lag.

I later learn that in my ability to keep working, albeit duly compromised, I am lucky. Most sufferers are rarely able to continue working at all, even from home. Many experience a state known as brain fog, an inability to focus on anything, which consequently renders even the most sedentary work impossible. They cannot concentrate on reading, on watching TV. Some are too tired to shower, to make it to the toilet by themselves.

My fatigue seems only to express itself in my outer shell, the bones, the muscles. My mind is still firing, still overactive. The copy I deliver is unremarked upon by editors (this is a good thing; they mostly only respond to complain), and when I finish ghosting the memoir, the book finds a publisher. The fact that I am able to work at all is something I do not take for granted.

By the third week of July, school is over, and my relief is considerable. Now I have no reason to go out at all. I can just rest, rest until I am better.

'It's not good for you, staying in all the time,' says Elena, concerned.

I agree with her, of course, but every time I go out now, I come back catatonic. It is the most unsettling sensation. It scares me. I tell her that I am simply responding to what my body appears to be telling me: stop. In truth, all I want to do is retreat, be by myself. Because I'm clearly no good around anybody else.

The start of the summer holidays feels like torture. Amaya thrums with an energy I can see radiating off her. She cannot understand why we are not going out. She is used to me taking her everywhere, on the bike, on the bus, the train, to shops, playgrounds, to the lions in Trafalgar Square, Hamleys. But now here we are in the kitchen, and now in the living room. For a change of scenery, we will perhaps go up to my room so she can play Mathletics on the computer. She is bored. She wants to go swimming, to the zip wire. She wants a play date, ice cream.

One afternoon, we go on a trip to the corner shop. We are going to make cookies, Elena's suggestion, and for this we need eggs, flour, sugar, things to sprinkle on top. Her excitement is propulsive, and she pulls my hand as we walk along the road and round the corner, saying faster, faster. The corner shop to me suddenly feels like an exotic foreign land. I used to visit daily, but now haven't in over a month. It is not the same man behind the counter but a different one, a stranger. He nods hello. We find what we need, then I go to look at the newspapers, which as ever are cruelly arranged the wrong way round, upside down, to deter loiterers like me from browsing. We go to the till and pay.

It is on the way back that I feel it, the dizziness, the seeming solidifying of muscles. Inside me, something is flaring, then melting, oozing into a gravitational pull. Suddenly I am furious. This is ridiculous. All of it, highly illogical. I do not understand it, and I refuse to accept it. I can't, I won't. *Pull yourself together!*

I look down at Amaya, at her bright smiling eager face, urging me home, into the kitchen, into aprons: big cook, little cook.

We make a triumphant mess in the kitchen, flour everywhere, broken eggshells in the mix, Amaya laughing, jubilant, eager to learn; my beautiful little girl with cake mixture stretching her smile from ear to ear. But the whisking proves my undoing. I don't seem to be able to summon the strength.

'Shall I do it?' Amaya asks.

I find the strength now, as a matter of urgent necessity, and so I whisk and whisk as required, completing it only because I cannot face a five-year-old's disappointment.

We arrange the cookies onto a baking tray, one blob bleeding into the next, then we slide the tray into the oven. We now have to wait for a quarter of an hour. I suggest that Amaya goes and watches television. She does, and I promptly curl up into a ball on the kitchen floor, vibrating with a tiredness that feels like a viral attack. I want to fight back, but cannot. My mind spins wildly. What is happening to me? How can I make this stop?

Soon, Elena is taking the girls to Spain to visit family, and leaving me home alone for 14 days. She wants to cancel, to stay with me, but the truth is I cannot wait for them to go. I am not functioning as either husband or father, and their daily presence is a painful reminder. Perhaps alone I shall feel more equipped to . . . to what, exactly?

I don't know. All I know is that I will miss them terribly, but that I need the solitude, the quiet, the brain space to start to begin to digest all this.

But then, a day after the cookies, the elderly next-door neighbour turns visibly yellow and calls for help. I see him being stretchered into an ambulance, to hospital, never to return. His son, arguably wayward, definitely drunk, is his sole beneficiary, and just a few days later takes possession of the dilapidated semi-detached house attached to ours, which he promptly transforms into Party Central.

And so all that prospect of peace and quiet: gone, vanished, just like that.

Four

The first time I see him is through the living-room window. I am not spying, though venetian blinds can sometimes give that impression. He is striking: big, bulky, of indeterminate age, mid-30s probably. Bald, unshaven, fag in mouth, a photofit stereotype writ large in his England shirt, forearm tattoos. He is carrying a corner-shop plastic bag, red with white stripes, not a Bag for Life by anyone's standards. A six-pack is distorting its shape to breaking point.

There had never been noise from our next-door neighbour previously, and only now do I realise that this was due not to some very solid brick soundproofing but rather to the fact that he was a quiet man. A sound comes through the wall now, the *kchww* of a can being opened. Then the TV, blaring. Presently, an operatic belch, which sets a pattern for the rest of the afternoon: the constant burble of the television, a succession of *kchww*s, a great many burps.

He drives a van, white, but doesn't seem to work. Whenever, still not spying, I see him pass my window, he is returning from the corner shop, another red-and-white-striped plastic bag struggling to keep hold of its contents. He likes to stand in the concreted-over back garden smoking a cigarette and shouting into a mobile phone. Often, he sounds angry.

Friday nights, he hosts parties, post-pub things, half a dozen new friends, more. No music, just a lot of talking and arguing and laughter wafting through the walls. It's like the walls aren't there at all. The noise permeates my house, up the stairs and into my bedroom. Around two or three in the morning, I become aware of an acoustic guitar, somebody giving a passable rendition of 'The Drugs Don't Work', then 'Wonderwall'. I check the glow of my alarm clock, and figure that things will wind down soon. They don't. I toss and turn, and drag my pillow over my face.

It is gone four now, so late it is almost early. If he is lucky, and he often is, a woman stays over, accompanying him to the bedroom whose back wall is shared with mine. My new neighbour is a silent lover, but she, whoever she is, has taken note from pornography. Her orgasms are laboured and screeching and, I am sure of it, faked.

I begin to have fantasies in which I wield baseball bats, no mercy shown.

The Friday-night parties prove popular. They begin to start on Thursdays, sometimes Wednesdays. They go on until Sunday, occasionally Monday, even Tuesday. They go on all night. They never get too raucous, there is never the thump-thump-thump of heavy bass, just the constant hum of people drunk, stoned and, later, wasted. In the mornings, someone will stumble into the garden and vomit enthusiastically by the shed, then return to the kitchen for more. Occasionally, night bleeds into day and nobody notices, 'The Drugs Don't Work' serenading my protein-rich lunch. Occasionally things get ugly, mostly with the women who extend their parameters of tolerance for one another until they cannot, at which point they start screaming, one a cunt, the other a fucking slag, and it spills out into the garden where the men separate them with placatory offers of cigarettes, one each.

When my family comes back from Spain, it is Elena who goes to complain. They greet her warmly, offer apologies and invite her in for a drink, a drag. But they are forgetful, and careless, and cannot regulate their volume. We begin sleeping/non-sleeping on the sofa bed upstairs in my room and experimenting with earplugs, and waste hours online looking for houses in different parts of London, different parts of the country, preferably detached, with a moat.

In time, my pacifist wife begins to share my fantasies. She too wants a baseball bat to wield with impunity.

For the two weeks my family are away, despite the racket next door, I retreat into a shell I didn't even know I had. The house becomes my hermetically sealed cocoon. I barely go out. Days are slow. Each morning I spend a couple of hours writing, then head downstairs for a change of scenery, sit on a chair and read. Occasionally, mindful of my new protein needs, I boil an egg for a mid-morning snack, which, if nothing else, helps pass the time. The heating of the water takes three minutes, the boiling of the egg takes four. Eating it is a regrettably swift business, and 30 seconds later I am back in the living room, on my chair, finding my place in my book. Every little thing I do I make last as long as I can, so that later might come sooner.

There is little work. It is summer; everyone is away. The ghosting project is all but finished, and I am delaying the gruelling editing process, because while I am bored, I'm not *that* bored.

The sun is out —it is by now late August, so sunshine is no guarantee — and I sit in the garden and breathe the air. The neighbour has a friend around. The friend has a dog. I make my way upstairs to the girls' bedroom window to peer: a Staffordshire Bull Terrier, a malevolent grimace to its Joker grin.

Mid-afternoon seems to drag towards a permanent standstill. It is too early to watch TV, and I have done all the work I can do for one day. Two hours until dinner; what to do? I have a hot bath filled with Epsom salts, Epsom salts another condiment believed to be helpful for those fatigued. Absorbing the magnesium is said to be good for the muscles, which is all I need to know. By now I view my body as a kind of petri dish upon which to attempt all manner of experiments in pursuit of health restored. I am so used to all the daily vitamins that I no longer need to be reminded which to take when. I have come to loathe the application of the so-called Magic Minerals, but I continue to apply them every morning just in case. Almost everything I am doing now to this end is *just in case*.

Dinner, delivered on Monday morning by Ocado and a rare opportunity for human contact, is health-conscious, and unaccompanied by wine. It is evening now, so I can watch TV without feeling awful about it. Before sitting down, in the dark, to watch the Danish noir I am by now addicted to, I go out for My Walk. This essentially comprises my entire daily exercise regime, but to call it a 'walk' is exaggeration. Because the slightest exercise outdoors has swiftly rendered me worthless this past month, I find myself becoming helplessly fearful of it. So the walk is minimal, and quick, my destination each night the postbox just off the main road around the corner. To get there, in a pair of trainers so unused of late that they almost revert to being new, I have to walk out of my door to the end of the street, turn left at the corner, and then up to the main road. I am never good with measuring distances, but let's say it's 10 parked cars. Now I am at the main road. I take a left, walk on a little further, then stop, look both ways and cross the road. Then the postbox, which I touch ceremoniously. Now return.

I am back on my sofa within four minutes of having left it, a journey that once would have taken me 30 seconds. The sofa is still warm. I switch on the television as the exhaustion goes about its curious business, like streams of cigarette smoke, or the liquid in a lava lamp, extending into my muscles and tendons, perhaps even the cells, and weighing everything down with the tenacity of quicksand. It is hard to believe that the legs that have taken me to all sorts of places for the previous 40 years now find it quite so difficult to do something quite so effortless.

I am in bed by 10. I would take drugs to sleep but 'The Drugs Don't Work' will only wake me up again by midnight, and then again at two, at three.

Morning comes early, and I am still carrying the fatigue from last night's outing to the postbox. It will take almost 14 hours until I feel ready, mentally and physically, to dare to repeat the journey again.

When the next-door neighbour is at last fast asleep, face down in all likelihood, then I suppose it is true that, in addition to my solitude, I have my much-craved peace and quiet. Elena suggested I might try meditation while she and the girls were away, another recommendation she had come across that sufferers can, and often do, benefit from. Dolittle had suggested similar. I browse it online, and come across something called yoga nidra, a sleep-like state of meditation. It isn't easy dismantling all of the long-held prejudices I have harboured for anything remotely New Age, but needs must, and so I cue up a 35-minute practice on Spotify, click Play, and assume the correct pose on the floor, on Elena's yoga mat, arms by my side, eyes closed.

I have never meditated before, nor ever seriously considered it, despite encouragement, and sometimes outright pressure, to do so. I had grown up with a mother who was very New Age in her outlook. She did yoga in the '70s, and was vegetarian at a time when such a thing was viewed with deep suspicion. She cooked meat for me only reluctantly, and while friends got crisps and chocolate snacks in their school lunch boxes, I would get chicory and celery. In the late 1980s, as I was finishing with education and getting ready to leave home, she became increasingly committed to Tai Chi, then quit her job in order to give herself over to it entirely.

After I developed repetitive strain injury in the early 1990s, she felt she might be able to help. I had already made my position clear on Tai Chi, that it was not for me, and so she recommended instead I try the Alexander Technique, which teaches people to better align their bodies, to sit properly and learn to relax the muscles and ease the otherwise perpetual build-up of tension. She felt this would help correct my posture and, theoretically at least, ease the pain, which was constant. My reaction was a knee-jerk derision long fostered by a diet of TV comedy and playground mockery that poured scorn on anything that lay outside of the limited realms of what passed for ordinary. Everything New Age was funny because it was claptrap, all yoga and falafel and open-toed sandals, and so all too easy to laugh at.

I had laughed at my mother too, and only agreed to some Alexander Technique after my NHS physio, a professional, corroborated it as a good idea. 'Ideally you'd have done this years ago,' he added, 'and if you had, you wouldn't be here now. But it can't hurt. Go.'

My mother found me a practitioner not far from where I was living at the time, in the bedsit-laden backstreets of Shepherd's Bush. She was an older woman in her 60s, who worked out of her soft furnished living room in Holland Park. She opened her front door dressed for comfort in loose grey and black cotton, a magnificent mane of grey hair flowing past her shoulders and down towards her coccyx. She wore open-toed sandals, in March, and this was all I needed to reinforce every prejudice I had.

She beckoned me into the front room, where three other people, in their 20s and 30s, were sitting. They looked up expectantly at me and nodded hello. I sat, and noticed a very particular smell in the room. It emanated from the floor, where four dogs lay, each fast asleep, two on their backs, their four paws pointing to the ceiling, genitals proudly displayed.

I remember little of the hour I spent in the lady's company, and I could hardly have guessed that, 20 years later, I would be spending many more countless hours taking similar instruction from people who knew better than I did on matters of health. I do recall that she spoke at length about the importance of posture, and how many of us today carried ourselves poorly, and so no wonder we were all in so much pain. What*ever* did we expect? She got each of us, in turn, to walk in a straight line before her, and then to sit on one of her dining chairs, for assessment.

'You,' she said to me, somewhat coldly, 'are a lost cause. Where do I start?'

I was out of all alignment, apparently. I carried myself too much on one side. I stooped. The speed of my gait aside, I walked like an old man.

She scolded each of us in turn with a schoolmarmish exactitude. The dogs didn't stir. I elected not to go back for a second session.

My mother was disappointed, but not surprised. She then suggested I go and see a holistic masseur, a friend of hers from Tai Chi, who might also be able to help. Because she knew I'd say no, she had already paid for my first session, and we both observed strict rules about wasting money. He lived in a small flat in Pimlico, and was expecting me one Wednesday evening at six.

The door opened to reveal a youngish man, perhaps a decade older than me, in jeans and a waistcoat, hair tied back in a pony-tail. Everything about him was gradual: his movements, his gestures, his smile, the length it took him to open his mouth and finally offer me not just a curious smile, but an actual 'hello'.

Because I wanted to see only the negative in him, I became immediately suspicious. This kind of inner calm, this quiet radiance, I decided in my 23-year-old wisdom, could only come from someone whose soul had been spuriously saved by a religious organisation.

His shelves were booklined with spiritual titles. There was an acoustic guitar in a corner of the room. It was a small room, and became, at one point, a kitchen. He asked me to disrobe, then to lie down on the massage table he had positioned by the curtained window. A candle was burning. He asked if I would like camomile tea.

When he came back bearing two mugs, I was wearing only boxer shorts and my T-shirt.

'Should I lie down?' I asked.

'When you undress, yes.'

Reluctantly, for it was cold and I was shy, I removed my T-shirt.

He pointed to my briefs. 'And those?'

I wanted the look I gave him to be challenging, even combative. But all I felt was a helpless timidity. 'Is that really necessary?' I asked.

He smiled. 'You have a problem being naked?' The question was rhetorical. 'This is interesting. Perhaps we should talk about this first.'

Like the Alexander Technique woman, this was two long decades ago, and I cannot claim to remember precisely how I remonstrated with my mother afterwards, but I do know that I did remonstrate, forcefully. She kept her recommendations to herself after that. Over the ensuing years, my mother herself was open to all sorts of alternative paths. She never remarried after my father left her, and carried with her a lingering depression that reignited whenever she saw a romantic film, or read a book by Anne Tyler, or spent more than a week in the company of her parents. She was forever seeking a kind of peace that proved stubbornly elusive. Still a strict vegetarian, she frequently dabbled with veganism, but didn't eat very much of anything at all. Secretly, she was anorexic, and had been bulimic too. Even before the cancer, she was skin and bone. She renounced traditional medicine in favour of self-reflection and St John's Wort, which meant no longer reaching for the Nurofen when she had another of her headaches. The headaches proved resistant to St John's Wort, and so she suffered in silence when I wanted her not to suffer at all. She delved deeper into the world of Tai Chi and the people she found there. I loved her very much, and always felt protective of her. The inner peace she craved was nothing I on my own was ever going to help her locate.

There developed a clique within her Tai Chi group. Instinctively, she tried to resist it, wary perhaps. There was something insidious about it, the inner circle treating the outer with deadpan mocking, these interlopers, city workers mostly, who felt they were attaining true spiritual calm simply by attending an hour a week, then heading off to the pub. The authentic disciples gave all the hours they could, irrespective of licensing hours; they made sacrifices. The course leader singled my mother out. He said that she had potential. She was increasingly invited to stay back after those from the outer circle had left. She started to practise every day, at home in the morning before work, and at the centre in the evening after work. Having grown tired of her secretarial job, she quit, insistent that she could live frugally, and she devoted all her time to the practice of this most graceful, and meditative, martial art. She became strong, with solid stomach muscles and arms like steel. She seemed almost happy, and I was happy for her.

The inner circle became her soulmates. Some of them lived together in a latter-day commune, but the house was in ill repair in a part of East London still years away from regeneration.

They encouraged my mother to sell her tiny studio flat, the proceeds from which could be put towards a much larger place in an undeveloped part of Hackney. They could all live together, and practise Tai Chi every day.

My mother was a very trusting, giving woman, the most generous person I have ever met, and she hated that she sometimes felt suspicious of the inner circle, and of how they may have been taking advantage of her. She voiced her worries to me, and of course I played to type, pouring scorn on them. I told her to tread carefully, to follow only her heart.

A few years later, when she was dying of cancer in hospital, the inner circle chose not to visit. She accepted their reasons implicitly, that hospitals and hospices had negative energy. At her funeral, only a couple of them turned up. They gave me a lift to the Tube station afterwards. On the way, I said that I hoped my mother would have liked the service I had spent so many nights agonising over. One of the inner circle gripped my arm tightly. 'Oh, she did. She liked it very much.'

Really? I asked. How did she know?

A kindly, benevolent tone to her voice: 'She told me.'

Yoga nidra, says Wikipedia, is a 'sleep-like state which yogis report to experience during their meditations. Yoga nidra, lucid sleeping, is among the deepest possible states of relaxation while still maintaining full consciousness.' It is an ancient Indian tradition, linked with spirituality, and is believed to purify the unconscious mind.

Distinct from yoga itself, then, which is more the adoption of specific bodily postures, it sounds pleasingly narcotic. There are plenty of yoga nidra meditations on offer on Spotify, and choosing between them is easier than I would have anticipated. Though one guided meditation is much like the next, its success for the individual rests entirely in the detail: what is said, and the manner in which it is delivered. If either are skewed, then the whole thing tumbles like Jenga blocks, and I can no longer concentrate on silencing my mind because my mind is too busy poking fun at their spoken inanities, or else correcting grammatical mistakes. The pedant in me rarely lies dormant.

'Take in a deep breath in,' one tells me. This infuriates me: why two *in*s? It's either, 'Take a deep breath in' or 'Take in a deep breath'. 'Take in a deep breath in' annoys me the way Paul McCartney annoys me when he sings about 'this ever-changin' world in which we live in' throughout 'Live and Let Die', thereby rendering the whole thing null and void.

'Imagine yourself as a single drop of water floating in a warm sea,' goes another one, American, and I imagine a Californian woman with unbound hair, a translucent dress and weight issues. 'You are one of billions of drops that make up a vast ocean. You are just one drop, but one of many drops, all of them just like you. You float on the surface of the ocean, glistening in the sunlight. You float in the mid ranges of the sea, affected by currents and tides. You float in the depths, the deepest reaches of the ocean, where it is still, and dark.' There is a pause of 20, maybe 25 seconds. I think she has gone, before suddenly she comes back. 'Become aware of the one who witnesses the one who floats in the ocean,' she continues. 'Become aware of the awareness that you are not just the one who is aware, but also the witness of the one who is aware. Turn your awareness on your own awareness.'

Several of the American-voiced meditations I come across reference money issues. 'A lack of finances; bad credit', as one puts it. I never come across money issues in those given by Brits or Indians, and the Indians are clearly the masters here. It is the Indian accent I am most drawn to. I love the melodic rhythm of their voices, the lulling properties of their vowels . . .

Over many long minutes of meditation, I find I have all the time in the world to mull over things like the lulling properties of vowels.

The first time I do yoga nidra, a couple of months after the diagnosis, I wait until nightfall, convinced the darkness will help me prepare for a more easily accessed meditative state. The practitioner I find, Anandmurti Gurumaa, has the most wonderfully calming voice I have ever heard. It is soft as expensive toilet paper, three-ply, while behind her what may or may not be a sitar seems to experience an elongated bowel movement. She tells me, in her clipped English, to lie down on my back with my palms turned upwards and to adjust everything, my body, my clothes, until I am completely comfortable. She suggests that during yoga nidra, which she, with her greater experience in such matters, refers to as 'yog nidra', no 'a', there should be no physical movement. I should be completely still.

The moment she says this, my body is assailed with phantom but entirely real itches: my nose, my forehead, my ears, first the left, then the right. My belly button, my balls, the arches of my feet.

It gets ridiculous, and so I get up, click Anandmurti back to the start of the practice, scratch everywhere one more time, and begin again. 'Lie down on your back with your palms turned upwards,' she says again in her soft chocolate voice. 'Make a resolution to yourself now that "I will not sleep, I will remain awake throughout the practice". And be very sincere. Just listen to my voice.' The *v* in her voice coming out as a languid *w*.

She tells me that I must not intellectualise or analyse her instructions, something I will be accused of doing many times by many other people in the months and years to come. 'Be very attentive. And if thoughts come to disturb you from time to time, don't worry. Relax; bring about feeling of relaxation in whole body. Be still. Develop your awareness of the body from the top of the head to the tips of the toes, and mentally repeat the mantra: ommmmmmmmmmmmmmmmm.'

As with so many things we experience for the first time, I consider all this improbably fantastic, a revelation. Just a few minutes in, and Anandmurti is blowing my mind. I am in a mental bubble bath.

She suggests I make my resolve. It has to be simple. I am to say to myself a short, positive statement, 'whatever you wish for yourself: good health, spiritual life, self-realisation. *Samadhi*.' I have no idea what *samadhi* might be, but later find out it refers to a higher level of concentrated meditation. I say my resolve – 'I have overcome fatigue; I am returning to health' – three times, and goosebumps chase themselves up my spine and tingle tightly across my scalp. It is the most exquisite sensation.

She now tells me to concentrate on different parts of my body, the right hand, the little finger, the forefinger, the third, the ring, the thumb. 'Be aware.' Then the palm of the hand, the lower arm, the elbow, the upper arm, the shoulder, the armpit, the right waist, the right hip, the right thigh, the kneecap, calf muscle, ankle, heel, the sole of the right foot, the top of the right foot, the big toe of the right foot, and then, one by one, each of its siblings.

'Don't try to concentrate,' she says, which confuses me because I have been concentrating on each of these parts of my body, and likely frowning as I do so. 'Just be aware.'

Then she switches to the left-hand side of the body, the hand, the fingers, the arm, above the waist, below. She flits from one body part to the next, busily but calmly, methodically, while the sitar continues to wail in low-level intestinal pain in the background. I feel heavy, pleasingly so. Occasionally an itch does come, but I override the impulse to scratch.

Anandmurti moves up to the head now, the forehead, both sides of the head, the right eyebrow, the left, the space between the eyebrows. Helplessly, my thoughts drift to Liam Gallagher in the video for Oasis's 'Whatever', and how he doesn't have any space between his eyebrows. Anandmurti moves on, and I quickly refocus. The nose, the tip of the nose, the upper lip, the lower lip, the chin, the throat, the right chest, the left chest, the middle of the chest, the navel. The whole of the right leg, the whole of the left, both legs together. The whole of the right arm, the whole of the left arm, both arms together. The back, the buttocks, the spine, the shoulder blades. The whole of the front, the abdomen, the chest.

'Now total body together. Full body. Now, once again, we will rotate our consciousness. Right toe, left toe . . .'

My mind alights on each part of my anatomy as she draws attention to it. I am even heavier now, sleepy. 'Don't sleep; remain attentive. No movement at all, the body remain still.' And mine really does. I am flushed with pride. *Look!* I want to cry out to the empty house. *Look at what I'm doing!*

She says that my body is lying on the floor, and that I am floating above myself, looking down, seeing it from head to toe. This feels empowering, somehow. Almost exciting. I have never done anything like it.

She wants me to concentrate on my breathing. Not to force it, merely to observe, to maintain my awareness. Complete awareness. But I cannot now not force it. The moment you become aware of your breath is the moment you helplessly begin to control it. But it doesn't break the spell, and the breathing is stronger now, coming from deeper down. I can feel the rise of my ribcage, my stomach inflating and deflating like a balloon. Complete bliss now. It is all distinctly otherworldly, and a little weird, but good weird. Her voice remains utterly hypnotic.

She wants me to count my breaths from 27 down to one: 27 navel rising, 26 navel falling, 25 navel rising, 24 navel falling. And so on. I find this unexpectedly difficult, being required abruptly to perform a task where moments before I was merely being led. I recognise irritation, and want to speed up my breaths if only because the very act of counting backwards is spoiling the deep plateau of peace I had so recently been in the midst of.

A moment later, she is talking again. There are no numbers in my head. I search in vain but find none. Had I fallen asleep? My mouth is dry. The sitar is distant, but still there, its one long note stretching doggedly towards infinity. My head is woolly: 27 navel rising, 26 navel falling, 25 navel rising, 24 navel falling.

There is just the sitar now. Where has Anandmurti gone? Will she speak again, or does the sitar never end? Shall I sit up, stop?

'. . . Now stop your count, and shift your attention to your chest.'

She's back, telling me to be aware, that my chest is rising with each breath, and that I should be, and remain, aware. And then she starts to count.

The counting again. I am bored of the counting, and don't want to do it any more. I do the counting: 27 chest rising, 26 chest falling, 25 chest rising, 24 chest falling.

'Say the words and numbers mentally to yourself,' she says. 'Be aware.'

I am aware. I think I am aware. I get all the way down to one, then start over. My ribcage feels the effort of it. I see, in my mind's eye, the bones lifting and separating, my diaphragm a slow-motion trampoline.

'Stop your counting,' she says, and I feel irritable again. I had been on 8 chest rising, 7 chest falling. There were only six to go. This sensation of uncompletedness does not sit easily with me.

Now there is a visualisation exercise. She will name things, and for each I should develop a vision of them on, she encourages, 'all levels': feeling, awareness, emotion and imagination. If I am unable to do this, she adds, 'no hassle'.

She begins. Over the next few minutes, she moves through burning candles, endless desert, torrential rain. Snowcapped mountains, sunrise and sunset. Birds flying across the sunset, a

canvas of white clouds. Blue sky. A Buddhist smiling. She tells
me that I am walking on green grass, that tall trees are shading
me, that I am approaching a temple. A dim light glows from the
temple. I reach it, and place my right foot on the step, and then
the left, and enter a courtyard.

I want to know what is in the courtyard.

'Now you are close to the door, and you see inside . . . *the
temple*. There is a beautiful image of Shiva.'

I do not know who, or what, Shiva is. The name is familiar,
but how am I to develop a vision if I don't know what, or who,
Shiva is? *No hassle*.

She says that the image of Shiva is beautiful, sitting in the
lotus posture.

Lotus I know, or think I know. It's some kind of yoga position. Something cruel to do with the ankles touching the tops of
the inner thigh.

She mentions red roses in front of his statue.

His. I had imagined a *her*.

'Bow down to Shiva.'

No, I find myself thinking.

'Close your eyes, and you are feeling immense joy,
immense joy.'

As she says this, 'immense joy, *immense* joy', in that beautiful voice of hers, something unexpected happens. A waterfall of
pinpricks washes over me, drenching me, and where moments
before I had felt heavy, now I feel light as air. The sensation is
full-bodied, euphoric.

'Now is the time to repeat your resolve. The same resolve
which you did in the beginning. Do not change it, and repeat for
three times, with full awareness and feeling.'

'I have overcome fatigue; I am returning to health,' I say to
myself, and repeat it three times. The goosebumps are not fleet-
ing. They remain.

'You have awareness of your body, from the top of your head to the tips of the toes, and say mentally in your mind: ommmmmmmmmmmm. Once again: ommmmmmmmmmmm.'

I hum and thrum. My neck, my chest, my wrists, the backs of my knees — all pulse. I can feel my heartbeat, the rising and falling of my stomach. I am aware.

'Stretch your body, do not be in a hurry. Move your fingers and toes. Slowly sit up, and now open your eyes.' A pause, then: 'The practice of yoga nidra is complete.'

It is as if I have woken from the deepest, most refreshing sleep. Yoga nidra has been around for centuries, I later read. Where has it been all my life? I feel amazing, invigorated, curiously whole. Perhaps this is the key I have been looking for. I resolve, right here, now, to practise every day, twice a day, so desperate am I to revisit those sensations. And, with it, to get back onto the path towards health, and to get better.

I will go on to do yoga nidra many more times over the next few months, and though I am always calmed by it, and rested, never again will I achieve quite such a spectacular natural high.

This of course leaves me utterly bereft.

Five

The long summer changes me. I enter it one person and emerge at its conclusion quite another, life slowing down emphatically and turning me timid, afraid, a coward. I learn to view my fatigue the way David Banner did the Incredible Hulk: terrified of angering it lest it unleash its full force and rage. At home, negotiating my way slowly over three floors, I am more or less fine: tired, yes, always tired, but in a way I can cope with if I don't think about it too much. Survival instincts kick in: as long as I am okay here, within the house, on hand to help look after the children, to cook for them and play with them, then I will settle for that. Just grant me that, I whisper to myself as if in prayer. The merest excursion outside, however, depletes me in ways I still cannot fully comprehend. The shortest of strolls is now enough to sap me of everything.

I become alert, too, to every twinge of weariness, every possible warning sign, that tingling calm before the storm. In this way patterns are being created. My brain remembers. I am putting up limitations in pursuit of self-protection, unaware of the vicious cycle I am entering into. Because the more scared I remain, the more adrenalin I produce, and the adrenalin uses up what limited reserves of energy I have left.

And so I develop an expertise in micro-management. I place myself under house arrest, and rarely leave. This is hard for many reasons, the least of which is that it's not *that* nice a house, it's not big enough, not comfortable enough, and I grow bored of my confines quickly. Every day is the same old bedroom, bathroom, living room and kitchen. If the sun stays out for long enough, I dare to venture into the garden, but no further.

School starts, the autumn term, and Evie enters Reception. Elena takes the girls to school in the morning, then leaves work three hours early in order to pick them up again. Her boss is not happy with this situation, and neither am I. Their arrival home is a low point. They come bounding in, discarding scooters, bearing smiles, and Elena hugs me, asks how I am feeling, then disappears upstairs to my office, her office now, to make up for time lost. To offset feelings of emasculation and shame, I busy myself with the girls, feeding them snacks, helping with home-work, officiating over TV, breaking up squabbles, counting star jumps on the trampoline. They know nothing of what I am going through, and I love them for their ignorance. The more I am around them, the less time I have to feel sorry for myself.

Still, I hate that Elena has to do this and also that her boss, a woman I have never met, knows that there are now *problems at home*. My instinct is to tell no one about this, but as the months go by, and in the absence of extended family, Elena needs to rely from time to time on the help of friends and neighbours, as well as work colleagues. All are kind and concerned, and they talk to Elena about how I am doing behind my back. On the rare occasions we all meet, we stick to polite conversation only: house prices, sport, the weather.

Most nights, I cook dinner. If the fridge is empty, Elena stops what she is doing upstairs and goes to the shops, but everything else I make sure I do: the cooking, the washing up. Afterwards, Elena comes into the kitchen to tidy up all the things I've missed.

Bedtime is a high-energy ordeal, but I insist we stick to our rota: one night I do it, the next night she does. By seven in the evening, I am all but worthless, and the hour it takes to get the girls up the stairs, into the bath, onto the toilet, their teeth brushed and pyjamas retrieved from under the bed depletes me in the same way a 10-mile bike ride once did. By the time it's done, both of them in bed and still wide awake, with still so much to tell me, I make my way down the hall into my room and collapse onto the mattress. At some point, I will make my way beneath the covers, but not yet. Elena comes to visit, her empathy a painful underlining of my helplessness, and then I sleep a dreamless sleep and awake 10 hours later if anything more tired still. I resist sleeping in the day, for that way madness lies, and instead count off the daylight hours until mid-evening, when the idea of crawling back into bed at least seems permissible.

It is the weekend that offers adventure, two days when I allow Elena to cajole me – 'for your sanity,' she says – out into the world. These are events that require meticulous planning in order to minimise the physical effort required. Ten footsteps from the front door to the car, a short drive to the playground that has the shortest walk from its car park. Then a bench on which to sit, rooted to my spot. If the girls want pushing on the swings, carelessly located at the far end of the playground, Elena gets up to do it. An hour later, back in the car. Rather than returning home just yet, a pit stop to Costa or Nero for coffee and cake, a little more diversion, another change of scenery. Once in a while, I am rash and daring. I see a bookshop on the way home, and ask if we might stop. Elena double-parks and I get out, on my own, suddenly walking from here to there, into the shop, breathing in its smell and luxuriating in what are to me, by now, novel surroundings in both senses, going upstairs to fiction, downstairs to biography, all the while fielding texts from Elena warning that a traffic warden is lurking and that the girls are getting restless, and so I cut short the visit and come out with a bag full of books, full of apology and the most sincere gratitude.

I pay the price for this afterwards, however: for the next few days, I am David Banner at his most remorseful, several fathoms beyond mere ordinary tiredness, and always bemused by it, shocked and distraught.

As the autumn progresses, Elena is beginning to despair on my behalf. The most restive summer of my life has not alleviated my symptoms at all. If anything, they have settled in and become habitual, the new norm. I have tried to fight the condition – with strength and reason, and the application of coarse minerals – but this does not seem to have worked, and the fear now overrides everything. I am passive towards the condition, not active. If asked, I tell Elena I am waiting to start to feel better, then I will do more. But she argues, reasonably, that if I don't take steps towards that myself, it might not happen.

'You never go out any more,' she says. 'You're becoming agoraphobic.'

I reel at the very suggestion, like a punch to the stomach. I cannot possibly be agoraphobic. How can I be? I simply have a fear of this all-too-real fatigue, which seems to be evoked through physical exercise alone. I can manage the level of physical exercise in here, but I cannot out there. Does this make me agoraphobic?

I went to have a haircut the week before, preparing for the excursion via Journey Planner online, a faintly ridiculous thing to do for a two-mile round trip, but grimly necessary now. It involved taking a bus to a nearby barber's, the bus empty save for a few elderly people on the way there, and packed on the way back with schoolchildren. It had felt good to be somewhere else, to talk to somebody other than the television screen. The young man who cut my hair had tattoos all over his arms and neck, of Dracula, Frankenstein's monster, Munch's *The Scream*. He told me that the world was ruled by the Illuminati, a group of elite leaders and celebrities who control all aspects of our lives. 'Look at 9/11,' he said in purported explanation. He told me that Barack Obama was a member, and also Kanye West, Rihanna and Beyoncé, and said that it would be obvious to anyone who had met them, who had shaken their hand. I told him I had met three of the four he had mentioned but noticed nothing untoward. The barber gawped at me, then took two clear steps back, just in case.

I arrived home feeling good. I didn't like my haircut, of course, he had cut it too short, but it would grow back. I judged the expedition a success until, an hour later, it revealed itself a failure. By evening, my insides were ash. I had no appetite, no strength, and craved sleep. It would take five days to recover.

While waiting it out, life is happening elsewhere, without me. I am no longer actively searching for much work, I go nowhere, my social life has stopped. Elena is doing everything for me, which makes me feel guilty and ashamed. I want to take control, to fight this.

But how? I still do not know where to turn. Breaking my no-googling rule, I find myself researching Dr Dolittle a little more, only to read more bad things about him, more letters of complaint, and so he is ruled out as a potential salvation. Besides, there is a four-month waiting list for his clinic. I need help now. *Now.* I can see no point in returning to my GP, who will only refer me to him again. My sole option, then, is the DIY approach, to throw myself into whatever private therapies, treatments and programmes I can find. All I need is time, patience and money, none of which I currently possess in sufficient quantities.

With the post-pub disruptions from next door ongoing, which our insistent complaints do little to stem, I decide, first, to focus on my sleep. I am reading about the importance of rest, and how to do it well. Sleeping properly, not lightly, but deeply enough to release sufficient levels of dopamine, is important to everyone, but crucial to someone with depleted energy reserves. I am now mostly using yoga nidra to fall asleep to, and though Anandmurti Gurumaa had implored me to 'stay awake', other practitioners have less of a problem with dropping off, some even actively encouraging it. We by all accounts continue to listen on an unconscious level that never sleeps, like a light that never goes out. And so every night I fall asleep to body-rotation instruction, visualising my fingers, my toes and Shiva, whom I have since googled – undeniably a boy, but a pretty one.

To my surprise, I do not tire of yoga nidra, but rather become accustomed to, and even reliant upon, it. But I do find myself wanting to supplement it with something else, something that either goes deeper, or perhaps resonates more. You can only really throw yourself into things by employing a scattershot approach, I decide, and so the logic I employ is this: the more I try, the more enlightened I might become.

I come across an audio meditation practice called LifeFlow, the conjoining of the two words presumably designed to illustrate the effortless link that should exist within all of us in the ideal world we wish to inhabit. It promises startling results.

'You can allow this scientifically proven audio technology to bring your whole life into perfect harmony and feel peace of mind today!' reads the website blurb, employing, as these things do, a proliferation of exclamation marks in the hope of encouraging, or at least fostering, belief. 'YES!' it goes on, peremptorily, 'please give me instant access to this break-through technology.'

It is hard not to read such bold and hectoring claims without arching an English eyebrow at it, not least when LifeFlow, as far as I can make out, is essentially meditation muzak. It offers a free sample, eight minutes of it, during which time 'happy' endorphins and anti-ageing hormones should by all accounts flow through my mind and body. I will start to feel creative, it promises, my brain will feel revitalised, and the new thoughts I shall, as a direct consequence, experience will emerge from my 'hidden subconscious genius within'.

I had not previously given much thought to my subconscious genius within. I hadn't even known I possessed one. All I wanted was for my sleep to be deep and restorative. The first downloadable CD, which comprises 40 minutes of meditation soundtrack, retails at $67. This, I learn, is merely an introductory soundtrack. There is more. The complete 10-CD boxset goes for $977. But I am lucky, because I happen to be visiting the website at a time when they have an offer on, and so it is currently $777, and comes with a one-year money-back guarantee. By signing up to this, I will also qualify for further CDs on things called Optimal Learning, Creative Flow and Discover Meditation as FREE GIFTS (their capitals), which, it is claimed, have a retail value, despite not being available in the shops, of $331.

It is here that I hesitate and take a step out of myself to observe things objectively. I am walking a narrow line that divides being desperate to get better and merely being desperate. I am not the latter kind, not yet, and so I find it hard to believe that $777 will buy me not just renewed health but also on tap creativity and intelligence, even though I would love to believe it because, frankly, I could do with a bit of both. But I do listen to the '8 Minute Wonder' sample, and I like it, a babbling brook busy with the sounds of rapidly running water, chirping crickets and windchime effects. Through earphones, the sounds bouncing from one bud to the other and pouring directly into my brain with such urgency they temporarily render all exterior thought impossible, I find I am transported into another world that is vivid and bright and alive. I revisit the '8 Minute Wonder' several times over the next few days in pursuit of meditative top-ups.

It is during my prevarication that the emails begin.

'How about that LifeFlow demo track? Awesome, isn't it?' it reads by way of introduction. A lot of bold print follows. It wants to know how it made me feel, whether I became soothed and relaxed. Most people do, it assures. But the email reveals a little anxiety, too. It worries that I might not have listened to it yet, and if this is the case, then 'you absolutely must'. It promises me that I won't regret it, that I'll be converted, and swiftly - so much so that I will want to upgrade, at the previously mentioned cost, for something called the 'Industrial Strength' version.'

The email is signed, in an inky scrawl, 'Michael'. This is Michael Mackenzie, the man behind Project Meditation, a Scot who has lived in America for the past 30 years. He is, as I will come to find, terribly persuasive.

For legal reasons, I should perhaps state that I'm not suggesting Michael Mackenzie is a huckster. In fact, there is strong suggestion online of the effective science behind his efforts. There is corroborated argument that LifeFlow does decrease binaural carrier frequency, which places a temporary stress on the brain, which in turn causes it to grow, much like a muscle would. Many people who have signed up, I read on other websites, rave about its properties; as is the way with these things, others do not.

The next day, inky Michael emails again. His written approach is not a million miles from that of a used-car salesman convinced that the likely customer merely needs the bolstering effect of his italicised enthusiasm. He writes that, while he may not know me personally, he knows that I am someone seeking peace, less stress. I *want* to meditate, he knows I do, but I've encountered hurdles. I might have tried other meditation courses before, and come away disappointed. But this one, he says, is better. I alight on two words, in capital letters: 'JET FUEL'. He writes about the science of his methods again, and of the 'immediate and lasting rewards'.

'The next day, another email, this one telling me that doctors around the world were using the programme. He quotes two of them, extolling the meditation's myriad virtues. The tacit suggestion here is that if it's good enough for medical practitioners, it's good enough for us, too.'

After the flood, the deluge.

More emails, more bold type, more caps lock. FACTS and RESULTS always win over claims, he suggests. I choose not to read the FACTS and RESULTS he goes on to list, because life is short and I need the loo, and there are only so many bold and capital letters you can read on screen without feeling headachey. I click away.

Still more follow, each wheedling and cajoling and coaxing, Michael dangling his carrot, pinching and prodding, beckoning me ever closer, or at least trying to. It is when an email arrives asking whether I ever feel like I am alone, that I've no one to talk to, that no one can relate to my situation, or cares enough, that I feel the snap. This is the last straw, the camel, the broken back and everything else. If I had ever felt inclined to transfer him my $67, or even my $777, then this email ensures I will never do so now. Michael Mackenzie is becoming an email pest. Go away, I want to say to him.

I am at a low ebb, evidently, because, unusually for me, I decide to vent my frustration by playing him at his own game. I email him asking why he isn't giving me the time to come to my own informed decision about his offer, but is instead constantly badgering me. 'Does this really work on people?' I ask him.

I regret the email the moment I send it, aware of the futility of it, and, besides, who am I to complain about his salesman tactics? He is simply trying to make a living. But just half an hour later, a reply comes. Not from him, but from a minion, a terribly courteous woman who apologises for the hassle, insisting that badgering is not their intent; they merely want to make me, and everybody else, aware that their product is powerful, and just possibly life-altering. As an olive branch, she sends me a link to the first CD, worth $67, for free.

I am immediately chastened, and feel rather foolish, but grateful. I would be lying if I didn't say I was just a little excited, too. Weeks of his boastful emails have, it seems, had the desired effect. I have apparently, despite myself, bought into his claims, because what I am feeling now is close to anticipation.

It is a weekday afternoon, and, with the neighbours still sleeping off the previous night's excess, the house is quiet. I download the CD onto my iPod, then go out into the garden and sit on my new reclining chair, a recent present from Elena, and every middle-aged man's dream. Tilted back, glasses off, earbuds in, I press Play. It begins, the familiar babbling brook, the chirruping crickets, the distant wind chimes, each individual sound wonderfully resonant in the left ear, the right ear, both ears at once. To begin with, it sounds not merely similar to, but exactly like, the '8 Minute Wonder' sampler. And it is. It is the same thing, albeit with better sound quality, stretched over 40 minutes.

Nevertheless, it does sound wonderful, and its hypnotic cacophony holds me rapt. It is invigorating, and mildly hallucinogenic. But after repeated listens, I register no significant mental improvement, nor creative, nor anything else really, and so I cannot concur with, nor claim to find it as revelatory as, the people quoted on its website proclaiming just how much it has improved their lives.

LifeFlow does not change my life, nor its flow, but it does provide some meditative calm during torturously slow afternoons. At night, it helps drown out that other cacophony bleeding through the walls of our house from the partying neighbours next door.

And for that, inky Michael, I am grateful.

Six

It is at around this time that I start to keep a diary. I resist the idea at first, convinced I have little constructive to say on the subject. Besides, the idea of not just living it but recording it for posterity, on the page, seems to me depressing, almost perverse. Why catalogue such self-involved misery? But Elena says it might be a good idea; people have said as much on the forums she browses at night. And so I give it a go. They are sketchy entries and, once typed, never re-typed, never re-read, until now.

Elena will be proved right, as she often is: each entry serves, much later, as a reminder not just of how bad things got, but also of my mindset at the time. Reading those early entries now, written 10 months after I became ill, four months since my 'diagnosis' sent me spiralling, I barely recognise myself. I had thought I was dealing with it all with patience and stoicism. The entries suggest otherwise.

OCTOBER 3
I go out with the family to the park for a picnic, on the assumption that a bit of fresh air would do me good. Walked barely 10 minutes, but arrive home exhausted, the muscles in my arms and legs so heavy. I can barely move, unable to put the kids to bed. I hear them asking Elena, What's wrong with daddy?

OCTOBER 17
In bed by nine last night, completely wiped out. Awoke unrefreshed at 6:30, scarily exhausted everywhere, in my legs, my back, my

mind. My ribs ache, even my cheekbones, though surely this isn't possible? Too tired, I think, to work today.

Elena can't pick the girls up from school later, she has a meeting. I have to do it. I'm not looking forward to it.

Two hours after school pickup: horribly shattered, deflated, completely without energy. It tires me out just to sit down, even. Bad day.

OCTOBER 20

Another broken night's sleep due to the neighbour. I want him dead, a car crash, overdose, an accident — nothing that can come back on me. Playground with the girls this afternoon, and another painful reminder of my situation when Evie needed the toilet. There is a public WC on the far side of the park, beyond the football pitch. Find myself measuring the distance, and immediately deciding it is too long, I can't do it. But she needs to go. Is four years old too young to go by herself? Wracked with anxiety. In the end, Amaya takes her, and I stand and watch them, helpless, hating myself, tearful.

OCTOBER 25

Birthday. Too preoccupied to even consider the onset of midlife crisis. A good thing? Elena takes me to a nice restaurant, by car. The walk from the car park to our table is long, and I fret. Then I fret because the toilet is on another floor, down a long corridor. Still in denial, because I think to myself: is this all really happening? How could I let something like this occur? We order champagne, just a glass each. Couldn't afford a bottle anyway, but I still can't tolerate the alcohol, each swallow making me nauseous.

The only thing keeping me sane is work. Day to day, I check emails ('Hi Nick, hope you're well'), and am now busy editing the ghosting project, which is progressing steadily. This requires of me little more than sitting at my chair in front of my PC, and

I'm good at doing that. Elsewhere, the majority of interviews I do are on the phone. One time, an eminent writer comes to my kitchen for our assignation. I offer him coffee and biscuits, then more coffee and biscuits, and am so grateful *he* has come to *me* that I can see he has difficulty in extricating himself from my clinging company two very long hours later.

This was highly unusual. Nobody else visited my kitchen. The journalist travels, not the talent. And because telephone interviews are never particularly fulfilling, I must travel still, irrespective of the complications in doing so. Public transport is beyond me right now, and so I settle for the bespoke, door-to-door services of a taxi firm.

I spent very little of my previous four decades taking taxis anywhere. They were the preserve of the wealthy, I thought, or the financially carefree, and I was neither. I knew of some people who claimed they had expense accounts, but expense accounts were like the Loch Ness monster: often talked about, rarely seen. I had always managed quite happily on buses and Tubes; now it's chauffeur service. For a few minutes, I marvel at the prospect, the sheer extravagance of it, the comfort, the space, the leather upholstery. It is a sophisticated way to travel.

Not by minicab, it isn't.

But if nothing else, travel by minicab is never dull, and in some respects I have more adventures in the back streets of Norbiton, East Putney and Old Street, in a dented Nissan driven by a displaced Iraqi with dissident leanings, than I ever did in Mumbai, Lima or Havana. A perpetual clock watcher, I am never, not ever, late for a job. I would always factor in potential delays, just in case, then arrive considerably early but happy to potter about until the appointed hour. I do not have such flexibility with minicabs. They have a mania for being early, perfectly understandable of course, but this means they deposit me at my destination early, which leaves me standing aimless, and restrictively tired, on a street corner waiting for the time to catch up with me. The journeys there are always complicated. The driver has little English and a lack of knowledge of his immediate surroundings. He relies a little too heavily on his satnav, which cannot help but seek out the capital's most congested streets. We stew in traffic, which encourages conversation, and over several months I hear the fascinating and terrible stories of exiles: the man whose extended family are lost in Tikrit while his wife is ill at home in Hounslow, and whose children are unruly and talking back to him in the 'English way'; another, from Zimbabwe, who regales me with happy tales from his Rhodesian childhood before we narrowly avoid being crushed by an oncoming lorry to whose driver he bunches up a fist and shouts, shrilly, his voice suddenly scaling an octave, 'You . . . you *bully!*' The driver from Afghanistan who grew up in Berlin and hates his native country and everyone in it; and the other who tells me that America will pay dearly for George W. Bush's actions in the Middle East for generations to come. I am, he says, to mark his words.

Occasionally, I am late, the traffic's fault, not the driver's. One time I am later than I have ever been for a job: 90 minutes. I was supposed to meet a much-loved character actor in his central London bolthole in the morning. By the time I arrive, it is afternoon. I run up the two flights of stairs and into his house, past his PR's pained expression, and I shower him with apologies, pulling the shirt away from my neck to allow the flopsweat to pour unheeded. He takes one look at me, sits me down on his couch and opens a bottle of champagne. I don't have the heart to tell him I currently have no tolerance for alcohol, and so I down two glasses.

It helps. In all sorts of ways, it helps.

NOVEMBER 1
Another bad day. Waves of tiredness, repeating over and over, leaving me incapable of anything. Spent the whole day waiting for it

to pass, Epsom salt bath at seven, bed by eight. Yoga nidra diffi-cult only because it's hard to make positive affirmations, and believe them, when you feel so catastrophically tired after so little exertion. I'm trying to understand all this until it seems explicable, reason-able. But I can't, and it isn't.

NOVEMBER 4
Awake by dawn, good sleep, but tired still. Mid-morning: increas-ingly lethargic, despondent, and really quite spectacularly shattered. It's mental and physical now, because I'm aware I feel very low. Five months in, and instead of seeing even the slightest improvement, it's just getting worse. Evening: absolutely awful, unspeakably tired, but I insist on putting the girls to bed. They notice nothing awry, climbing all over me before demanding I read one book, then another. I love them for it.

NOVEMBER 11
Low. The tidal wave of tiredness that comes so promptly the moment I step out of the door makes me fearful of stepping out the door. Catch-22. Was Elena right? Am I agoraphobic? I hope not. Couldn't cope with that, the shame. Elena, I know, is having a tough time adjust-ing to all this, and seeing her struggle makes me realise how serious it is, along with the imperative to DO SOMETHING. Later: Despite still being dreadfully tired, we manage sex. It felt like a necessity, a reminder of before.

I start to look into low-level exercise. 'Relax,' Dr Dolittle had told me. 'Do some yoga.' I have certainly relaxed these past five months, often to the exclusion of everything else, but I have not broached yoga. Perhaps now it's time.

Elena buys a DVD. It is presented by two people, one a preposterously muscled and unreasonably good-looking man whose face is a masterpiece of learned serenity, and the other a pretty woman from breakfast television. Together, on yoga mats, they work through a series of elaborate and elastic poses. The backdrop is idyllic, a Greek island in the summertime, all shimmer and haze and distant olive groves. I try to follow along, but struggle. The DVD purports to be for beginners, but the pair are clearly experts, with a penchant for showing off. After an initial introduction, they whip through pose after pose with an impatience my former self would have recognised, and approved of. 'Quicker now,' he says, downward dog, having previously taken a languorous 30 seconds, now over and done with in 10.

As the DVD progresses, it is difficult not to become aware of the sexual chemistry between the instructors. It becomes so heady – to me at least, a man possibly seeking distraction – that I have to pause the DVD to google whether they are an item. My findings prove inconclusive. Either way, their frisson makes me envious, and does little to further my *prana*. I continually struggle to keep up. His movements are fluid and graceful; his muscles ripple. Mine do not. I cannot do anything he can do, and he is doing it too quickly, and with too much preening confidence. I keep having to reach for the Pause button, because while he sweeps a foot back to join the other, and then up again, arms now on hips, arms now arching in a sun salutation, I am huffing and groaning, and not finding any humour in my predicament at all.

At the end of each session, I am exhausted. This is perfectly reasonable, because I am clearly unfit; it is okay to be tired after a yoga workout. And I am doing lots of it: the downward dog, the bridge, the shoulder stand, more. Blood rushes to my head, my thigh muscles stretch until they can stretch no more. I become short of breath, and have to lie for several moments on the mat beneath me in order to regain it. Is this really Yoga for Beginners, I wonder. It decimates me. It's too much. I can't do it.

So I switch DVDs, and order another one online, this one especially for people like me, fatigued. My instructors are Sue and Fiona, comely, kindly women, and between them they do the very gentlest sort of yoga. It lasts for about 40 minutes, and they perform their moves alongside a couple of students among whom they share absolutely no sexual chemistry. I am grateful for it. I still struggle with the movements, but I get progressively better at them, and each day I can manage stretches I could not manage the day before, which lends it all, for me, a slightly, but nicely, competitive edge.

It soon becomes the activity around which the rest of my day revolves. Soon I want to do it twice a day, but for what are very likely the wrong reasons: as if by proving that I'm committing myself so attentively to the practice, I shall get better quicker. That's how it works, right? No. It is still my instinct to rush in everything, and to rush my way through this, because I don't seem to possess the patience demanded of me by the fatigue. It isn't funny any more. I am bored of its disruption. My sleep patterns are deeper thanks to the meditative soundtracks, which claim to release serotonin and reduce cortisol, and I am now listening to something called Delta Isochronic Tones, which purportedly offer anti-ageing support, and to something else called Delta Binaural Beats, which encourage empathy and compassion, and also a deepening of spirituality. Each night, our bedroom pulses with aural activity, weird bleeps and electronic hums that only a Radiohead aficionado could truly appreciate.

But all of it, the yoga and the sleeping and the enforced patience, doesn't seem to be working. I am unaware of any significant changes for the better. As far as I can gauge, and despite my silent pleadings, it isn't having the slightest effect, any of it. I am furious.

Elena tells me to look at it another way, to appreciate that I am lucky, that I have crashed into fatigue rather than into something more serious, like cancer, an aneurysm. She is right, of course, and while I would never wish for a more serious illness, in my more morose moments I do nevertheless crave to be in the hands of a doctor with a plan of action. If I had had cancer, I'd have had chemotherapy by now. It would have either worked or not. The lump would be out, or else metastasised, but either way, *something would have happened*. With this, nothing has, at all. It is all so inert. I simply wait for change, and gently (ineffectually) try to speed up the change. But I still have no real clue what I am doing, and the long-term outlook seems bleak. This is not an illness in the strictest sense; there is little progression to it, no obvious conclusion. Life is grinding slowly down to walking pace – or at least it would were I capable of walking pace, which I am not.

Nothing is happening, no respite. I am 43 years old. I cannot possibly spend the next three decades like this. I need to do *something*.

I read about the early stages of CFS, and how sufferers should tread carefully: the body is still in shock, still majorly depleted of its natural resources. Anything too strenuous can have ruinous effects. I am soon to be reminded of this.

Winter is upon us now, and the girls come back from school with blocked noses and sore throats. I become fearful of flu, and so decide it makes sense to inoculate myself against it. One Saturday, we drive to a nearby Boots. The pharmacist questions me before the procedure, and as I answer, she frowns, and then strongly advises against it.

'My sister has CFS,' she tells me, her hand on my arm. 'She had a flu jab, and it wiped her out for months and months. She was awful. So you shouldn't have this; I'm not going to give it to you. Just go home; rest.'

NOVEMBER 18
Another broken night's sleep for all the usual reasons, The Drugs Don't Work, performed acoustically, at 3am, and repeated several times. Today will be the last day of the so-called magic minerals. There's only so many times I can rub damp sand into my chest without feeling

the fool. Fed up, too, of taking all these pills. It doesn't seem to make any difference, and the horse-sized ones always stick in my throat.

My early-morning yoga interrupted by Evie, who walks into the room and sits on my chest in the middle of the bridge pose. I battle on, but her sister joins her, and soon they are both alongside me attempting to do the downward dog, or trying to while giggling and pronouncing yoga 'silly'. Flashback to walking into the living room of my childhood once to find my mother mid-pose, and wondering what on earth she was doing, how strange she was . . .

For the rest of the day my whole body aches in tiredness and tightness. Everything feels like it needs unwinding, loosening, a good run, swim, ten miles on the bike.

NOVEMBER 20

A humbling realisation of my new cowardice: now I really am terrified of walking, of anything that might bring on another tidal wave of fatigue. The walk from the car to the café this afternoon — a few hundred feet at most — brought about the utter conviction that it was too far, that I couldn't handle it. By the time I was sat drinking my coffee, my body was sinking to the floor, a leaden weight. My head swam, total panic, freakout. Psychosomatic?

Bed by 8:30, catatonic.

NOVEMBER 21

25 minutes of the yoga DVD, including pre- and post-breathing exercises. Difficult, tiring, but in a good way. The ache in my stomach muscles continued well into the evening. Because of the yoga? All this self-obsession! But I'm no longer able to take my body for granted as I once used to. Everything I do carries freighted significance.

Later: The neighbour's motorbike has just burst into flames, and was completely burnt out by the time the fire brigade arrived. So some good news, then. Ha.

Seven

Nobody else knows; they've no idea. This is my secret alone, albeit one I must reluctantly share with Elena. And it's a shameful one. I feel ashamed of what has happened to me, of what I have somehow allowed to occur. I still feel I could have prevented this, though quite how I'm not sure: by being stronger? More Teflon-like? But my sense of self has been destroyed these past few months; I am not who I thought I was. I've travelled so far from there to here, and so quickly. It's all too intangible a condition to share with anyone and expect them to fully understand it when I still don't understand it myself. And so I keep it a guilty secret.

If friends come to visit, I can act as normal around the kitchen table as anyone else, and if they notice I'm not drinking, they don't mention it. When we visit friends, we drive, even if they happen to live two streets away, because how else am I to get there? But this makes things awkward. When we are visiting friends who live two streets away, I don't particularly want them to see us arrive. They'll think us lazy, or else spectacularly unconcerned about our carbon footprint. So I insist that Elena drops us off, as quietly as possible, near their front door, then quickly and covertly parks around the corner before we ring the bell together, a ridiculous pantomime I cannot quite see any way out of. It is surely no coincidence that I become pronouncedly reluctant to indulge in any social activity whatsoever. All I really want to do is hide.

And those people who do know, those whom Elena has confided in, don't understand the true scale of it. They know that I am 'unwell', but it is clearly a vague, even mysterious kind of unwell, because I haven't been in hospital; I don't look any different. I'm not on crutches; my skin hasn't come out in blotches. I haven't shed weight; haven't lost my hair. I can hold a conversation the way I always did, and can laugh and joke as normal. In company, I have learned to conceal it well. I don't want anyone's sympathy or pity, or, worse, their amused confusion. 'Wait, you're *still* tired?'

Elena tries to prompt me into direct, combative action, increasingly convinced that I have given in to the illness and retreated to such an extent that I might struggle ever to emerge from it. For the past few months now, our lives have shrunk exponentially, and everything we do is strictly regimented around my increasingly limited abilities. I walk nowhere now because I cannot. If the weather is fine, and Elena impatient, I might concede to accompanying them on a picnic, but it has to be on a patch of grass no more than two metres from the car. And while everyone else is busy strolling around or playing games, I will remain on my patch of grass, going nowhere. There are newly logical reasons for this. Every excursion now requires of me some mental mathematics. I have to assess the distance, the number of footsteps required of me, and then come to the helpless conclusion that it is simply too far, that it will take too much out of me. 'I don't have the energy' used to be a figurative phrase. Now it's a literal one.

The 'no known cure' taunt I'd read online has clearly had a profound impact. At some level, I already believe myself a helpless case. Life has changed so profoundly and so quickly these past few months that I cannot envisage things returning to the way they were. This is the new me now, and I must get used to it. But Elena, for one, doesn't want to get used to it, and worries that we have become a family that goes nowhere and does nothing. Recently, she told me that she was frantic during these months, distressed at having lost the man she had married, that she no longer fully recognised me, this helpless victim. She was fearful, too, for what we as a unit would become. Because what kind of life was this? And how sustainable, long term, could it really be?

After six long months, by now desperate for a plan of action, Elena comes across something called the Optimum Health Clinic (OHC). Based in London, it offers 'award-winning support for ME, CFS and Fibromyalgia'. When she shows me their site the following morning, I stall on the 'award-winning' bit, mystified that it is possible to win stuff for such things, but she insists I read on. It's an 'integrative medicine clinic with a specialism in the diagnosis and treatment of the condition'. It offers something called the 90 Day Programme, for which it is necessary to attend a three-day course at its HQ which, although the website boasts a Harley Street address, actually operates out of somewhere in North-west London. The course is expensive, £625, but the site claims that the total value of what is on offer – three days, a book, some CDs and DVDs – actually has a total value of over £1,000, and so the £625 in fact represents a 'massive concession'. It also offers a nutritional consultation, which it believes to be key in treating the condition successfully, at an additional £235, with follow-up appointments available at £125 an hour.

I am still doing the maths when Elena says, 'You should do it. It might help. And we've got to do something. We can't go on like this.'

I take a minicab there, and my driver is not happy about it. The journey takes us from one periphery of London to another, and we spend two hours crossing through endless congestion and many diversions. At one point, we nearly collide with a woman at a zebra crossing. It takes me a moment to realise the squeal of breaks I can hear is coming from this car. 'Fool lady,' he mutters.

Later, turning to me, which means taking his eyes off the road, something I would rather he didn't do, my driver says, 'You should be taking train. This is too far for cab.'

Architecturally speaking, given the disposition of its visitors, the Optimum Health Clinic boasts bad feng shui. It is a tall, handsome brick building located halfway down a quiet residential street, with a massive front and two potential entry points, one at either end, both of which can only be accessed by scaling a steep metal staircase. I ascend one, buzz, wait in the freezing cold for a reply, only to be told by a disembodied voice I am at the wrong door and need to go to the other one. When I am eventually permitted entry, I find another staircase, which I walk up slowly, puffing in a state of nervous anticipation.

I will be here for the next three days on what promises to be an intensive programme of information and instruction in pursuit of restored health and resumed well-being. For the first time, I am doing something proactive about my fatigue, in public, with other people. I set my phone to vibrate, then think better of it, and set it to silent.

The course is run by people who have had fatigue-related conditions themselves. Each of them has got better – in many cases, fully better. Framed photographs of staff members and former patients litter every window ledge, many of them featured in outdoor pursuits, in the wilds of nature, in walking gear, on bicycles, halfway up mountains. The message is blunt, but exciting and abundantly clear: *See? We are active and healthy again.*

I arrive, at last, at a large, high-ceilinged room, a long table at one end, next to a small adjoining kitchen, and at the other two large sofas in front of a whiteboard. Somebody, I do not catch her name but she is an OHC assistant, a former patient herself now training to become a practitioner, is on hand to make us herbal tea (strictly no coffee here, no caffeine), and to share with us her own journey from illness back to health. She used to be a lawyer. Now she is doing this. We fall into music talk, and she tells me she has recently been to T in the Park, Scotland's Glastonbury, and had felt tired but manageably so, and only towards the end of the third day. 'Had a fantastic time,' she beams.

She introduces my fellow attendees, all of whom had arrived earlier than me. There are six of us, five men, one woman. We are later told that this is unusual; it is normally more evenly balanced between the sexes. The six of us range in age. The youngest is 18, the oldest in her 60s. Two are students, and exceedingly shy. One is a former city worker, another in IT.

Introductions are awkward. Aside from the two students, it is clear that the rest of us haven't been in anything resembling a classroom – as this essentially is – in decades. We are a disparate bunch, and none of us really want to acknowledge, at least initially, the only thing we do have in common. It takes two cups of green tea before the former city worker, now in his 50s, comes over to talk to me. He is balding, and dressed in corduroys. His face and demeanour seem to me in perfect harmony, both full of an open friendliness and genuine warmth.

'So, how long have you had it?' he asks me.

I try to sound perky in my response, as if to convey to him that I shouldn't really be here at all, as if it's nothing major, nothing I can't handle. 'Six months,' I smile. 'You?'

He meets my smile, and raises it. He does seem particularly jovial. 'Oh, over 20 years now. You get used to it after a while.'

I flinch. I do not want to hear this, and feel almost angry at his presumption that I might. Who says I'm going to have this for 20 years? I turn away, on the pretence of filling my cup. I see the woman in her 60s sitting quietly by herself, tears pooling in her eyes. We later learn that she almost always has tears in her eyes, because she is always crying. 'It hurts so badly, you see.' She has had fibromyalgia, essentially chronic fatigue with pain, for decades. 'Most of my adult life,' she says.

I grow hot and uncomfortable. I want to leave. The realisation that I might be among my new peer group makes me shudder. If I could, I'd run. Tuning back into the collective conversation, I hear that both the former city worker and the man in IT play music, one the organ, the other the guitar. This conversation continues until the OHC assistant gently reminds us that it would perhaps be better to focus on the reason we are here. We laugh, but all of us feel chastened, and we settle back into a stilted silence. I fight the impulse to check my phone for messages. Out there, real life, normal life, continues without me.

And then Jess arrives, our practitioner, the woman who will lead us through these three days, and on into the following 87 of the 90-day programme as we make our way back to health, and to the point at which we too can send in photographs of our newly active selves in all-weather North Face gear.

Jess is in her late 30s, and is dressed for the office in white blouse, black skirt, modest heels. She was once a primary school teacher, a detail confirmed by her easy-to-follow manner, the way she makes eye contact, and how well she deconstructs complicated information into bite-size chunks for better digestion.

She begins by telling us that she too once had the condition, and that hers was so bad she couldn't leave her bed for months, her house for even longer. I notice that she is careful not to put a specific number on precisely how long, lest we use it as some kind of marker for ourselves. I am glad she doesn't. I don't want to know how long she was unwell, nor how long it had taken her to get better. Already in my head I have Dr Dolittle taunt: 'Could you afford to live off your wife's salary for a year?'

Jess says that, at her very worst, a trip to the bathroom for her was almost, but mercifully not quite, impossible. As she was the mother of two small children, her husband was forced to multi-task day and night, which took a toll. The former city worker nods in empathy. But she, Jess, is better now, and had felt so motivated by her recovery that she wanted to help others in similar situations. So she quit her teaching job and retrained as a psychotherapist specialising in ME and CFS cases. She tells us about the last holiday she went on, skiing with her family. The two oldest people in the room, who have suffered the longest, gasp audibly. Both have been ill for such a long time that Jess's ability to ski is greeted like a Lourdes miracle worthy of hallelujahs.

We are each given A4-sized folders whose cover reads 'The 90 Day Programme: Inspiration, Integration and Transformation'. It has a picture on the front of a woman in a red dress running carefree through a field, arms outstretched. Inside are maybe 150 pages of information, with chapters headed The Healing Zone, Your Body's Intelligence, Emotional Freedom and Beginning the Integration. I have not felt so daunted about reading anything since Mr Farrell insisted we finish *Moon Fleet* by the end of the week, a book none of us in second-year English had even started. We were to be tested on it. (I would get a C–.)

In front of us, at the whiteboard, Jess picks up a Magic Marker and starts to talk. On the sofa, I sit up straight. Beside me, the IT worker gives in helplessly to temporary sleep. The students take notes, the woman with fibromyalgia cries quietly to herself.

The term *chronic fatigue syndrome* is relatively new to science. It was first coined in 1996, but its general symptoms have history dating back several hundred years. In the 19th century, a neurologist called George Miller Beard, finding links between fatigue, anxiety, headaches, depression and even impotence, came up with the term 'neurasthenia' – 'a mechanical weakness of actual nerves rather than the more metaphorical nerves'. By 1955, doctors at the London Royal Free Hospital believed that the disorder was caused by inflammation of the brain and spinal cord, and recorded so many cases streaming in through their doors at that time that they considered it an epidemic, as if one might catch it like flu. By the 1960s and '70s, the symptoms were becoming more frequently attributed to a condition called chronic brucellosis (fever, malaise, tiredness), as well as to psychiatric disorders and depressions. It came fully into its own a decade later when it earned the nickname yuppie flu, and was widely, if ultimately erroneously, perceived to inflict high-flying city types in pressurised jobs, burning the candle at both ends and exploding somewhere in the middle. In 1996, in the UK, a report was requested into all the research to date, the results of which came up with the current label, chronic fatigue syndrome (often known by its acronym, CFS). Shortly after, in America, the Centers for Disease Control & Prevention recognised CFS as a serious illness, and in June 2006 launched a campaign to raise public and medical awareness. It now has World Health Organization status as a 'disease of the central nervous system'.

Invariably, as with so many newly identified illnesses, there is controversy surrounding the precise nature of it, both its cause and its subsequent treatment. The NHS's treatment of CFS is, according to many outside that institution, insubstantial. But the NHS stands firm. This is largely because, I am told, the traditional medical world works on a paradigm of medicine where one looks for specific individual causes of illness for which interventional treatment can be developed. So, for example, if you have a headache, you take a pill; if you have cancer, you undergo chemotherapy. There is no drug for CFS, and chronic conditions are always much more difficult to treat than acute ones because chronic ones have so-called multi-systems that affect the body in so many different, and frequently mysterious, ways.

When I speak to Alex Howard, the man behind the Optimum Health Clinic, he tells me that the medical world is still somewhat lost in regard to CFS because it doesn't meet the usual ways of understanding illness. There needs to be much more research into it, he says, but research requires funding, and funding is often predicated on unwritten guarantees of success. CFS is too cloudy an issue, too complicated to treat, to warrant much funding.

'But I would hope that in the next one to two decades that is going to change,' he says.

'One to two decades is a long time,' I say.

'It is, yes, but then these things do take a long time. It's much easier getting research money for things that have already been established. It is easy to get funding for, say, cognitive behavioural therapy [*CBT, which was pioneered in the 1960s as a way of conceptualising depression, and is now often prescribed as a form of treatment for those with CFS*] than it is for CFS.'

Chronic fatigue itself may be difficult to deal with, but the way in which we respond to it on an emotional level is much more straightforward. It is our very emotional responses to it that keep so many of us in the negative stress patterns on which it feeds. The fear becomes a difficult-to-escape loop, and the more evidence one builds up that physical activity prompts fatigue, the more the fatigue will follow physical activity. Before long, the sufferer is effectively brainwashed.

I am one of the approximately 62 per cent of cases whose fatigue was triggered after a virus. Many struggle to beat a flu, and many more had had glandular fever at some point in their lives. When I was 18 years old, and about to go to America for the first time, I was diagnosed with glandular fever. In the weeks preceding my departure, my glands had swollen, mumps-like, but the swelling quickly subsided, there were no other symptoms, and I felt fine. The doctor nevertheless told me to take it easy for a while. I explained that I was about to spend nine weeks in Pennsylvania playing sports from morning to night; the last thing I would be doing was relaxing. I asked him whether I should consider not going. His response was disarming. 'Ha ha!' he said. 'Good luck!'

Though Professor Peter White suggests otherwise, depression is commonly listed as the other major trigger in CFS cases, either of the chronic kind, or else circumstantial (i.e. prompted by a traumatic event – a bereavement, divorce, losing a job). And if not depression, then long-term stress, that most modern malaise which currently defines the 21st century perhaps more than anything else, is also a major factor. Recent figures suggest that fatigue now affects one in three people in the UK in some way, but this is widely considered to be an outdated figure. Given the difficulty over diagnosis, Alex Howard believes there are many more people whose daily lives are now consumed by an unexplained fatigue that they put up with until their body gives out. In many cases, it eventually will; for those whose bodies don't, there isn't much explanation as to why not. Some are simply tougher, more resilient, than others. It is reported that chronic fatigue affects three times as many women as it does men – although when I put this to other experts, the statistic is challenged – and that the average sufferer ranges in age from mid-20s to mid-40s. But children can also develop it, particularly students approaching exam time, and it can affect older people, too.

The fatigue itself presents differently from everyday tiredness. It is not eased by rest or sleep. It is easily provoked. The slightest physical exertion can result in the kind of exhaustion one might expect after running a great distance on little or no training. There are other related symptoms: many suffer from cognitive difficulties such as limited concentration (the aforementioned 'brain fog'). There can be poor short-term memory,

an inability to concentrate, and a general feeling of disorienta-
tion. Sleep can be problematical, either too little of it or too much.
There can be pain in the muscles (fibromyalgia), and recurring
headaches. There can be dizziness, nausea, palpitations. In some
cases, the individual might be capable of light domestic tasks
only; in severe cases, they are wheelchair-dependent, and can
be unable to withstand loud noise or bright light. Those who
weren't depressed before might find themselves depressed now.

There are moderate palliatives. Painkillers can be dispensed
to help with muscle or joint pains, and anti-depressants for
mood. But the sufferer must become expert in the management
of their own life in ways they likely never have been before.
They must manage their sleep better, their rest patterns, and
those who believe relaxation simply occurs the moment they sit
down will have to rethink their understanding of the word. Diet
plays an integral role, because the body uses an awful lot of its
daily energy resources on breaking down the food we introduce
into it. Caffeine is not encouraged, neither bread, nor too much
protein, too many carbohydrates, fatty food, fast food; heavy
meals in general. Pulses, lentils, nuts, soup, lots of fruit and
plenty of vegetables – all are great. Alcohol isn't.

Graded exercise therapy – which basically means extending
your physical exertions over time – is recommended by the NHS
and is considered the most effective treatment by those within
the NHS who treat it. However, this is contested by many of the
more vocal CFS sufferers, convinced it makes their symptoms
worse, not better. CBT is frequently employed, though it does
not cure the condition so much as help the individual manage the
symptoms and, more pertinently, their reactions to them. There
is much encouragement by all concerning that most loaded of
phrases, 'coping strategies'.

The internet is full of stories of people whose lives are
destroyed by CFS, while there are many self-published memoirs

from former sufferers whose lives have been turned around during their recovery process, and who have become evangelical as a result. Where once it was shrouded in mystery, now it is becoming increasingly everyday. Many people in the public eye suffer from it — actors, pop stars, television presenters, writers. Few seem prepared to discuss it publicly.

Ultimately, the sufferer must employ a largely do-it-yourself approach. They must investigate what is out there, and what works for whom and why, and how it might work for themselves. It's a big ask when we are so used to relying on the medical community for help when we are ill, and so initially the prospect is frightening. It can be a wretchedly lonely business, too. But over time, such an approach can start to seem rather empowering.

At the Optimum Health Clinic, they like to tell you that the first rocket to the moon, which did eventually reach its destination, was off course for 97 per cent of the time. At her whiteboard, Jess apologises for her drawing skills while sketching the moon, a rocket and a series of erratic dashes to convey its wavering path. 'But what this is supposed to show,' she explains, 'is that every time it did go off course, it course-corrected, over and over again.' She looks up from her drawing now, to make eye contact. 'The key thing to remember is that it got there.'

This will be the overriding message of these three days: do the work, and persistence will pay off. The course begins, and we start, naturally enough, at the beginning, with a discussion on chronic fatigue, the preconceptions and misconceptions, the limitations of the traditional recovery model, and how likely it is that what we have been told about our conditions to date by our doctors is wrong. 'ME/CFS/fibromyalgia is not a mystery,' Jess assures us. 'And when we learn to understand the way our thoughts and emotions impact on our body and our recovery, we can re-take control and create consistent results on our healing journey.'

The two students alongside me on the sofa make an earnest note of this, but it will take me several years to appreciate it, much less begin to act upon it.

Many alternative health practitioners find their calling because they once had cause to seek alternative health practitioners themselves. The Optimum Health Clinic was founded in 2003 by Alex Howard. Howard developed symptoms consistent with chronic fatigue shortly after his 16th birthday, and spent the next seven years searching out potential cures and remedies. Once fully better, he set up the OHC with a team of analysts, many of whom had also recovered from their own fatigue issues.

Howard is a ball of energy. YouTube footage of him, in which he discusses treatments and recent findings, reveals a man who can barely be contained by the chair he is sitting on. He gesticulates a lot, expresses as much with his face and hands as he does with his voice. You are left with the impression that he is someone who could beat you in a race by sheer determination alone. This is probably no bad thing for the figurehead of an organisation that aims to get you back your energy. He tells me that he set up the clinic as an antidote to the NHS's approach, which is still, in his view, more traditional, and unsuccessful. There is still a big mind/body disconnect in traditional medicine, he says, traditional medicine dealing with each separately, individually, but never together. Alternative therapy, whose genesis comes from the East, has always focused on the mind and body together. We would do well, Howard says, to adopt a similar approach.

'Chronic fatigue is burnout of the body. There are many different sources of that burnout, and many different variants, but it's basically a state where the body crashes as a result of too many different sources of stress.'

He says that stress and advances in technology mean it has become harder for people to fully switch off. The more we are stressed, the weaker our immune systems become, and so a lot of us are consistently tired for all sorts of reasons; they just haven't been labelled yet.

The OHC's approach is a holistic one, and it tries to get people into the right state to heal before they can go on subsequently to do just that: heal. It offers a selection of treatments Howard and his team believe have the most effect. Many of them revolve around breaking the negative adrenalin loop the stress has created. It offers no quick fix, but rather the slow process of self-solution.

'If you look at more established chronic illnesses like cancer,' Howard says, 'then there are many interventions for that on many different levels, and a lot of the research now is increasingly on the psychological and the emotional role in cancer, both in terms of stress being a causal factor but also in offering a better psycho-emotional support as part of the treatment in pursuit of better outcomes.'

His hope is that the OHC model will be adapted to these chronic illnesses as well. In the meantime, he is another niche practitioner in a growing field, and like all such people, is bullishly confident that what his clinic offers really does help.

I have heard of the fight-or-flight response before, of course, but have never previously given it much mind. As a species, we are programmed to pay more attention to bad news than good. This is purely Darwinian: survival of the fittest. We are designed in a way to look out for threat. Good news does not constitute a threat as much as bad news does, which is why the bad always affects us so much more than the good. This explains why, for example, we are so much more affected by criticism than by compliments.

Our beliefs, negative ones especially, can be powerful, more so if they are consistent with a threat. We are perpetually switched on for threat much more than we are for an easy, nice or even happy life. The genes that survive are the ones that are most attuned to potential danger, and so, in some sense, the more nervy we are, the more on edge, the more likely we are to survive. It is our emotions that dominate our lives, not the thoughts in our head.

But in order to remain healthy, we need to learn how to live a life without setting off those maladaptive stress responses. Too many of us live on adrenalin for too much of our lives, and so it is little wonder that eventually we become exhausted, mentally and physically, and that this makes us unwell.

All of us here are caught up in our fight-or-flight response, constantly creating more adrenalin than our bodies either need or, in their current state, can deal with. Jess illustrates this by talking about a caveman. When this caveman was out hunting, he often encountered sabretooth tigers. The default setting of any sabretooth tiger was hunger, his next meal – caveman, say. And so the caveman had to make an instantaneous decision: stay and fight, or flee? Adrenalin would help him ride out this situation, and frequently equip him with the necessary smarts to get away.

None of us are modern-day cavemen or women. We do not encounter such heightened threats in modern life, and so our responses do not need to be quite so alert or aggressive. But stress keeps us in this state anyway. We are doing what we can to survive, but we've got the maths wrong. We stress too much, and the more persistent it becomes, the less energy the body can produce, and so the more we begin, inevitably, to tire. Before long, the body enters into what feels like a permanent state of exhaustion. This means a rise in blood pressure, an impairment of the digestive function, a tailing off of energy production, and an increased susceptibility to infections and long-term illness.

This impacts everywhere – the body, the brain – and it grinds down each until, one way or another, metaphorically or literally, we collapse.

Understanding all this on a theoretical level isn't enough, says Jess. Just because we understand the point she is making does not mean we now have the tools to reverse such deeply ingrained habits. In order to even begin to heal, one must spend more time in a healing state than in a distressed state. If you have already spent time in a distressed state, then you have much work to do because the body is now convinced that everywhere lies threat. In some cases, each time you do something – walk to the park or from the bedroom to the bathroom, or attempt to complete some homework – the body creates a silent siren: *mayday, mayday*. At this trigger, the body produces adrenalin, which changes hormone patterns, which plays merry hell with the digestive function, which saps strength. Days, months and years can pass in this fashion.

The clinic recommends meditation, yoga, and also suggests we consider dismantling life as we know it in favour of new ways of seeing, doing, being.

It strikes me that there is a compulsion, not only at the clinic but in medicine in general, to separate everybody into absolute types. We are easier, as patients, to assist if we conform to a type. And if we have something like chronic fatigue, then it is also likely we are of a particular psychological type.

Jess is talking now about these types, and says we need to find out which one we believe we fall into. First, there is the Helper Type. This is someone who puts everybody before themselves to the extent that they overlook their own needs and end up feeling disconnected from themselves and from life in general. Then there is the Achiever Type, who believes that the only way to be accepted and loved is to achieve and succeed.

But the Achiever Type has difficulty acknowledging their own success, and so always craves bigger, better, more, the underlying fear being that without perpetual achievement, we – and life itself – are nothing. The Anxiety Type is someone who believes nothing is safe, that the world is in constant peril, a disaster movie made real, and that danger lies everywhere, on every door handle, every toilet seat, every turbulence-ridden transatlantic flight. Then there is the Trauma Type, a person who has suffered greatly in life, from the death of a loved one to a persistent illness, or who was perhaps the victim of an assault or attack and remained scarred as a result.

I sit listening to this with my friend in IT still asleep beside me, and the poor woman with fibromyalgia still weeping quietly in the next chair along, and I wonder which type I might be. I think I am too selfish to be a Helper Type. Jess explained that she was a Helper, and offered as an example the fact that she would often completely forget to feed herself while taking care of her children. I am very fond of my children most days, and I think I am fairly attentive to them, but I have never forgotten to feed myself. Elena later suggests I might be an Achiever, but the two students with me at the clinic are both Achiever Types, and they speak about the importance of getting A grades, and how anything less brings only shame and self-loathing. I rarely got A grades at school. And now I'm a freelance writer, a perpetually perilous profession I am not sure any Achiever Type would be quite so prepared to put up with. Which perhaps makes me an Anxious Type? I definitely have anxieties. I fastidiously check all foodstuffs in the fridge for sell-by dates, and ever since a friend of mine developed tinnitus I find myself turning the sound down on my iPod just in case. But I do not consider the world a dangerous place. Turbulence has never frightened me, nor the dentist's drill. I am also prepared to sit on public toilet seats if the need arises.

That leaves Trauma. When I was 21, as I was helping my mother move from the now-empty family house into a small flat, the large frameless mirror I was carrying to the removal van hit the front step, split and fell heavily, neatly slicing my right wrist an inch away from where I may have chosen to cut it myself if ever I wanted to try dying. The wound required 11 stitches, but I remember that the nurse was lovely, and calming, and that I was actually rather proud of the scar afterwards. So on reflection, I don't think this could possibly constitute Trauma. Later, when I have one-to-one counselling with one of the clinic's therapists, it is decided that maybe I have a kind of lower-t trauma after all, not because of the mirror, but because of my childhood in general, the product of divorced parents, a depressive mother, an absent father. The psychiatric world view, clearly, tallies with Larkin's. Later still, Elena will kindly point out to me my myriad behavioural tics, many of which, she believes, are redolent of Anxiety. The fact that I recognise myself in her description, despite having been blissfully unaware of them previously, makes me want to hold my head in my hands and howl.

Sometimes, Jess tells us, chronic fatigue might simply be genetic. After all, everybody deals with issues in their lives, and not everyone gets fatigue, do they? Just as not everybody who smokes will develop cancer, or have a stroke. Our genes do not necessarily have to determine the outcome of our lives, however. It is how we approach life itself, from a mental perspective, that counts.

All this information is new to me, and I have precious little idea how to navigate it. I sit in this room with my fellow patients, looking to all intents and purposes keen and thoughtful, but it is too much to take in in one sitting, and I am still not sure I should be here at all. The suggestion Jess makes — that we change so much about us and our circumstances as a matter of great urgency — is overwhelming. How am I supposed to go about doing that?

She stresses again that we need to be in a healing state. To do this, we must stem our overactive imaginations from lingering in their unhealthy corners, and become instead positive. This is not easy, and we shall have to work at it. We need to learn to recognise the very moment we start to run negative patterns in our minds. The point at which my own thoughts stray to my fatigue, she says, which sparks again the worry over it, is the point I need to challenge it, physically and audibly. I need to shout 'STOP!' and throw out my hands in a 'STOP!' fashion. I have to centre myself, to become aware of my hands, my feet, my breathing. Do this, and I will begin to learn to free myself of this heightened stress response. I have, too, to repeat some positive affirmations, to *see* myself better, unshackled from exhaustion and returned to health. These have to be vivid visualisations. 'Turn the colour up loud,' says Jess, 'and do it many times a day.' 'How many?' asks one of the students, Biro in hand. 'Ten,' she says. 'Twenty. *Hundreds*, if necessary.'

This seems unfeasible, and so we spend a lot of time now perfecting it, standing in front of the group and repeating our positive statements out loud, trying hard not to blush before our audience. It is all rather a rigmarole, but then this, I suppose, is the point. The brain likes its habits, and quickly reaches for them; to break them, a rigmarole is precisely what is needed, words and actions combined, and repeated over and over again, without a thought of how silly we might look or feel. This new territory comes with all new rules.

If this all feels fairly straightforward, a method of self-control I can at least theoretically appreciate, then EFT requires more of a leap of faith. This treatment, Emotional Freedom Techniques, has been described as a 'modern energy therapy', which presumably means it is not the kind of thing you should talk to your doctor about. It is claimed that EFT has provided thousands with relief from pain, disease and a variety of emotional issues. It is essentially acupuncture without the needles, whereby you establish energy meridian points along your body by tapping them with your fingertips while focusing on the problem. 'The cause of all negative emotions is an imbalance in the body system,' I read. 'Our unresolved negative emotions are major contributions to most physical pains and diseases.'

The internet tells me EFT is 'catching the attention of healers and spiritualists', which under normal circumstances is enough to put me off, and though the process may be a simple one, it is difficult to overcome a feeling of acute self-consciousness while doing it. It is methodically ritualistic: you stand and repeat the same affirmation you did during the STOP! process while manipulating a sore spot several inches above your left nipple (and it is referred to as a 'sore spot' because if you find it and rub it, it doesn't tickle). You then begin a process of tapping your body seven times on specific points around the body: the top of the head, the eyebrow, the side of the eye, under the eye, beneath the nose, on the chin, on the collarbone and under the arm.

It works by releasing blockages within the energy system, and it is these blockages that are the source of emotional intensity and discomfort. Such blockages limit beliefs and behaviours and the 'ability to live life harmoniously'. Emotional disharmony is believed to be a key factor in physical symptoms, and techniques such as this one are gradually being introduced within psychotherapy circles. Though its roots stretch back a long way, invariably to the East, it was created, and given its New Age handle, in the 1990s. Many practitioners report remarkable success, and it is said to be particularly good for helping to deal with anxiety, depression, insecurities and eating disorders.

What it seems ultimately to do is help you focus on an idea and reassess it. Jess says it has been a profound help to her in her recovery. She encourages us now to give it a go. After tapping, she says, we might feel that the problem has disappeared, or else reduced in intensity. Perhaps it – whatever 'it' may be – has moved to somewhere else in the body.

But my fatigue seems to me less specific than an 'it'. It's all over, so after I tap, nothing moves anywhere; I feel no different. I appreciate the intent, certainly: to look within yourself, to a deeper level than you have looked before. To take stock, to echo the literal breath with a metaphorical one, to change harmful thought processes, and to relax.

And it is relaxing, and I do it, over the next many, many weeks, because I am told to. While doing it, I ponder again on whether I am a particular Type, and whether some deeply buried denial is stopping me from seeing this, recognising it and working against it. I wonder again whether I might have depression. I do not believe myself to be the depressive type, but if I ever had cause to be depressed in my life, it is certainly now.

And so I go online and take a depression test.

Do you have difficulty falling asleep at night? reads the first question.

No.

How often do you feel tired and run down?

Right now, all the time.

In the last six months, have you gained weight or lost a lot (not due to dieting)?

No.

Has your sex drive become seriously diminished?

Not seriously, no. (Mercifully.) But diminished, yes, a little, because I am so often asleep these days.

Has a parent or sibling been diagnosed with a depressive order?

Diagnosed, no; depressed, yes.

Do you often feel like life is not worth living?

No.

How would you rate your daily levels of stress and anxiety?
In relation to fatigue, high; to everything else? Medium.
Do you experience delusions or hallucinations?
No.
Do you put on a happy face to hide feelings of sadness?
In company, yes.
Have you been through a recent traumatic event, such as divorce, death of a loved one, losing your job?
No.
Have you developed food cravings, particularly for carbs or junk food?
No.
Do you have suicidal tendencies?
No.
It concluded by saying: *If you have answered yes to at least half the questions, then you might be depressed.*

Though I imagine a doctor would conduct a more thorough test than a few simple questions posted online by God knows who, I take this to mean I am not depressed. But my mind undoubtedly resides these days in a perpetually anxious state, and so it is this I need to work on, in capital letters. STOP!

I am, initially, a diligent student. I STOP! all the time, dozens of times a day, though I never do quite manage hundreds, and I practice EFT frequently, but always privately. The self-consciousness over tapping parts of my body never quite recedes. Done alone in my room, I am fine; I go with it, hopeful and optimistic. But being caught in the act by a curious four-year-old does little to assist the positive affirmation on its way.

'What's Daddy doing?' Evie asks Elena one day.

In time, what I am doing becomes my 'thing', as in: 'I'm just going upstairs to do my . . . *thing*'. And if my daughters enquire as to what doing my 'thing' entails, I simply tell them 'work'.

My affirmation is always the same: 'I believe I am fully able to heal and recover'. I repeat it with as much sincerity as I can muster, but soon enough the repetition kills it, and the affirmation merely becomes repeated words. They start to sound empty, hollow.

On my third and final day at the clinic, I book the recommended additional appointment with the nutritionist. Nutrition is an important component to the maintenance of health, of course, but it is often hugely influential in the treatment of, and recovery from, fatigue-related conditions. My nutritionist is Tara, a lovely woman in her 40s, supermodel skinny, with long, flowing auburn hair and an appealing disregard for clock-watching. My costly session with her lasts an hour, but she is still asking me questions 90 minutes later. I point this out to her rather self-consciously, and she laughs. 'Oh, I'm always running over,' she says.

The sleepy IT guy in my group had recommended Tara. 'She completely changed my diet,' he told me in a manner I couldn't help but receive as a threat: his lunch now was pulses, his drink, hot water. But then the IT guy had already boasted about his previously poor diet of liquid lunches and late-night microwave meals. He had had a lot of wrongs to right.

Tara says that my pre-existing diet is fairly decent. My mother's lingering influence, I tell her. My formative diet was a belligerently healthy one. By the time I escaped her influence, first living with a girlfriend and then alone, I was cooking for myself on a Baby Belling, and forcefully rebelling. I had discovered Bernard Matthews' chief contribution to a hungry world, Turkey Drummers, which I ate with potato waffles, neither of which took up much space in my compact freezer. My 5 A Day invariably comprised cherry tomatoes, five of them. Or, if sliced in half before serving, 10. After a lifetime of granary and wholemeal, Mother's Pride was a daily luxury, and I had a week-end thing for pork pies, and, after drinking with friends, Chinese takeaways or KFC family buckets. Ben & Jerry provided dessert.

But by my early 40s, and laden with fatherhood, I happily fell under the influence of my far healthier wife, and back onto a diet of which my mother would have approved.

But Tara isn't about to give me 90 minutes of her time with-out making recommendations, and there are plenty. She wants to know what I have for lunch, my caffeine intake. She suggests I cut down on bread and eat more eggs, perhaps with rye crackers. Porridge for breakfast, or some wheat-free muesli. She insists on fish. I do not like fish. Pollock, she lies, has a far more gentle taste than other fish, like cod or tuna. She tells me to buy oatcakes, hummus. No more crisps, but rather nuts, seeds. Broccoli, spin-ach, kale. If I ever crave soy sauce, have tamari instead, which is wheat-free. Protein shakes are terrific, boosting the immune system and supporting the liver with antioxidants. Plain yogurt only, no more honey. For the past few months I have been spoon-feeding myself manuka honey, which promises antibacterial and energy-boosting qualities, straight from the jar.

'Yes, but what about your teeth?' Tara asks.

I stop buying manuka honey. Agave, she says, is a good sweet substitute. Think natural, organic. Replace Sainsbury's, even Waitrose, with Whole Foods, Food for Thought. Snack on pumpkin seeds, sunflowers, Brazil nuts, hazelnuts, walnuts, flax-seeds. Cut down on salt, sugar. 'And no more alcohol, at least for the time being. Think you can manage that?'

Towards the end of the clinic's three-day course, Jess tells us a joke. 'How do you eat an elephant? One bite at a time.'

It isn't funny, but then it isn't that kind of joke. Instead, it serves as a warning, reminding us that if we really want to get better, then we have to work at it. It is up to us.

As she wraps up, I suddenly feel genuinely fond of everyone I have come to know these past three days. We shake hands, hug and wish each other well. Jess encourages us to keep in touch, saying it is useful to touch base frequently, to be there for one another. And though we all promise to do so, none of us quite manage to.

Unless, of course, they all keep in touch without including me? (Classic Anxiety Type.)

When I leave the building, on a freezing Friday night, Elena and the girls are there to greet me. I haven't seen them for three days – incapable of the daily commute, I stayed with a friend who lived nearby – and I am so very glad to see them. Under my arm, I carry my folder, 150 pages I will have to read, then read again, in the hope that I have the mental capacity to take it all in.

'What's that?' Evie asks.

Truthfully, I reply, 'Work.'

The girls are hungry, so we stop at a nearby Pizza Express, me negotiating the walk from the car to the restaurant in my still customary maladaptive manner, stuck in a helpless fear that will keep me in a negative loop for many dark months to come. I order a pizza from what the menu promises is its new healthier range. It has a hole in the middle, into which is plonked a few leaves of lettuce. Less dough, new me.

The clinic's 90 Day Programme does not promise a clean bill of health, normality miraculously restored, after three short months, but merely greater understanding of a process that takes time, focus and patience. And so what looms large in my newly aware consciousness right now is the elephant itself, its size and heft, how immovable it seems, how indigestible.

Eight

DECEMBER 11
Still doing STOP!s and EFT. It doesn't feel any more natu-
ral, and still feels weird, but I surprise myself by being entirely open
to it, almost hungry for it. I do it as much as I can, always hopeful
and positive, and not, I think, cynical at all. Which surprises me.
Spent most of the afternoon watching the clinic's videos online, in
which they discuss how to get your head around the recovery process,
and also to maintain it – which clearly isn't as easy as it sounds.

The clinic's folder, stuffed with information crucial to my well-being, sits tauntingly on my desk, next to my keyboard, underneath a pile of books, CDs and magazines, an empty coffee cup and a small bowl filled with pistachio shells. Unearthing it, much less opening it, requires effort. I browse its many pages – Mental Conditioning: The Need for Repetition!, Working with Your Emotions, Restoring the Balance – and in doing so lose the will to read further. There are too many distractions: new books on my bookshelves, recorded TV programmes to watch. I want to spend time with my children. All of it appeals more, so the folder remains hidden, deliberately, beneath the desk mess.

In the folder's flyleaf, tucked into a little plastic pocket, are three pages of paper stapled together. These I do take out and read. They are headlined: *The benefits of meditation*. Since my first few experiences with yoga nidra I have rather let meditation slide. The pamphlet reminds me how it is a self-help tool crucial to reducing stress levels and inducing relaxation states, and how it can also be used as a gentle means of self-development. Meditation is a stress-buster, it triggers the relaxation response in the autonomic nervous system, which encourages the muscles to relax, digestion to improve and the heart rate to become lower, and also produces mood-enhancing endorphins while, at the same time, managing to quieten the stress hormones, the adrenalin, and all that cortisol, the steroid hormone released in response to stress. Cortisol increases blood sugar and decreases bone formation. In an ideal world, you want only to produce it in short bursts.

The pamphlet directs me to an online taster, and I watch a few minutes of guided meditation from a middle-aged woman called Linda Hall. Like Anandmurti Gurumaa, Linda has the voice and poise of complete tranquillity, and though I enjoy the experience, and also find that, at some instinctive level, I feel like I might want to practise meditation further, and go deeper, I am not ready, not yet, and so I click off. I am not sure why, and I do not articulate possible reasons, either out loud to Elena or to myself. All I feel, simply, is: *no*. Not for me.

I do not yet know that I will come back to meditation as my crisis deepens, and that Linda will become a soundtrack to my daily life. This is all still some way off. In the meantime, it appears that, despite the clinic's best efforts, I am at the moment my own worst enemy, and on a steeply downward slide. Things are becoming worse, not better. The fatigue deepens, and my resolve plummets. Were I to do that online depression quiz now, the outcome, I fear, would be different. I am lost.

And so I find myself reaching for something I had previously thought was strictly the province of Other People: therapy.

I have always rather secretly been drawn to the idea of therapy. I like talking to anyone who will listen, forever lumbered with a perpetual case of verbal diarrhoea. And, having spent two decades asking people often rather direct personal questions for my work and being intrigued by their responses, the prospect of finally answering some myself appeals, even if I have to pay for it. I am intrigued by what I might say.

Part of the clinic's 90 Day Programme is three follow-up conference calls, the six of us doing our level best not to talk over the other while Jess chairs the group dispensing advice and wisdom and support. It's a nice idea, but the calls always feel awkward to me, each of us reduced to disembodied voices on an uncomfortably echoing shared line, Jess often being required to encourage each of us gently in taking our turn to talk. Some report modest progress, others less so. One or two – usually the students – don't talk at all. At the end of one call, in response to something I have said, Jess suggests I stay on the line afterwards, 'as the issues you are having require, I think, some one-to-one attention'. A chill passes through me as she says this, and before the others leave, one or two wish me good luck. This does nothing to ameliorate my sense of unease or the oddly déjà vu feeling of being asked to stay behind by the teacher while everybody else goes home.

My problem is not a particularly difficult one to unravel: I am not getting any better, and I have proved myself all too easily influenced. The three days spent in the company of those for whom fatigue has become a miserable way of life have impacted on my Anxiety tendencies so propulsively that any Achiever characteristics have flown the coop. By spending time with fellow sufferers, I have seen my likely prognosis and come away convinced that it doesn't, cannot, end well.

Jess and I speak for another 10 minutes, one to one, teacher to pupil. She is kind and full of sympathy, and she concludes that I should have a few Skype sessions with her, each lasting an hour, each costing the equivalent of a flight to the sun on a budget airline.

The first session offers an uncomfortable revelation. I may well have been looking forward to what I might say in therapy – and by extension to what I might learn about myself – but my answers to her questions do not come easily. I had always imagined I would know exactly what to say in such a situation and that, given the opportunity to talk when I know that somebody is listening, it would prove difficult to shut me up. But Jess's questions are hard. She says abstruse things like: What is blocking you from returning to life? I haven't the faintest idea what she is talking about. There is nothing blocking me from returning to life outside of this illness, this condition. Is there? 'You tell me,' she says, and allows the expensive silence between us to stretch. A minute of not talking here costs me two pounds. I should not be focusing on this, the cost. And yet.

She asks those increasingly familiar questions, the ones regarding emotional fallout, bereavement issues, job difficulties, marital disharmony. What, she asks, is happening to me on a subconscious level? The answer to this last question is relatively easy and knee-jerk, almost a joke: I don't know, because it's happening on a subconscious level, isn't it? Jess tells me that all sufferers of CFS are battling something, some kind of trauma. What is mine?

I want to answer her, I really do. I think hard, aware that my hands and feet are becoming oddly cold. I want to conjure something up, a buried revelation, but fail. I um and er, my mind aware only that the clock is ticking. £30 already. I could buy three and a half books for £30.

Successive sessions mirror this pattern, and we skirt around the big, frustratingly elusive issue, neither of us making any obvious headway towards it. And so our conversations become circular and repetitive.

One time, she asks me: 'What if I told you you have to take a train tomorrow, for work – to Manchester, let's say. What would you say?'

The answer is instinctive, and I flush with embarrassment when I respond, truthfully: 'I'd say no. I couldn't do it.'

We speak once a week. It is always good to talk, and it does feel incrementally beneficial, but there is no breakthrough, and each session finishes with me feeling guilty for having made the previous 60 minutes so clearly frustrating for her. At the end of one, she makes a suggestion. She thinks it might be useful if I speak to another of her patients, somebody further along the recovery process. If I have reacted so badly to being around people still so mired in their own fatigue, then perhaps I would react more positively to those on their way back to full health. I like the sound of this, and readily agree. She says she will contact the other patient, a man my age, and an appointment is made for us to speak on the phone in a week's time.

It is, for me, a comparatively busy week. I have several commissions, and one morning travel to East London for an interview. I decide, in the spirit of taking things forward, that it might be good for me to go there by public transport rather than cab. The only way to confront my fears is to do so head-on. Elena drives me to the station, and I stand on the platform anticipating the train's arrival in a way I haven't before. I feel a thrill when I see it come snaking around the bend, almost like when my favourite band walks on stage. It arrives, the doors open, and I step into unexpected nostalgia. I sit in what had once been my regular space, the first set of four seats from the door. It is mid-morning, the carriage is mostly empty, and I have them to myself. I stretch out and, instead of reading, as I would normally do, I look out of the window, enjoying the view I had previously thought humdrum. Now it is novelty: the drab suburbs gradually becoming the city, the tower blocks, Battersea Power Station, the London Eye. I haven't made this journey for almost 18 months. I have missed it. Commuters get on and off, the train fills up, and I become reacquainted with the noise of other people's headphones, the sheen of their T.M. Lewin shirts, the backpacks so many are so careless with, bumping into heads and shoulders on their way out before the doors close, deaf to the mumbled complaints that follow in their wake. The adverts in my carriage are new, and on the wall by the door is a kind of barcode that we are encouraged to scan with our smartphones for access to exclusive content. Exclusive content to what? My five-year-old BlackBerry constitutes anything but a smartphone these days, and if it does have a scan facility, then this is a secret it has kept from me.

It is all so familiar, but so utterly new, the world moved on without me. Is this, I wonder, and not for the last time, what it feels like to be old – rendered outdated by youth and the march of progress? I arrive into Waterloo station to find much of it under construction, the M&S gone, so too the WHSmith, scaffolding everywhere, and I walk haltingly, self-consciously, in the crowd, to the nearest exit, where a pre-ordered minicab awaits to take me four miles east, to Spitalfields, where I interview a singer who tells me about her love of India. She makes me coffee and offers me homemade carrot cake.

She sees me off an hour later with a hug. 'I enjoyed that, it was like therapy!' she says, laughing. 'How much do I owe you?'

The sun shines, and life is good.

But then it happens again, on my way back, the familiar sensations creeping slowly up to smother me, to drag my muscles down. The cab that has taken me back to the station has stopped further away than I would have liked ('Too much traffic!' he shouts), and the walk to my platform is longer than any I have taken in over a year and a half. My body hums its curious activity through all eight stops, pins and needles and deep, deep aches. I try to remember some of Anandmurti Gurumaa's calming guidance, but summon up nothing. The train deposits me at my station, but at the far end, some considerable distance from the exit, something I hadn't thought about previously, because who in their right mind thinks about which section of the plat-form they will get off at? The ticket barrier seems miles away. I walk, because what else am I supposed to do? *Calm down, you fool.* But my body is no longer in control, or perhaps it's my mind, and so either, or both, conspire against me, everything I have learned in those meditation taster sessions gone. I'm all adrenalin and cortisol now, a lethal brew, and so whatever self-control I do possess puddles at my feet. It is all I can do to keep moving forward, to make it down the stairs, through the ticket barrier and out into the street beyond, where I flag down the nearest black cab and finally make it home, exhausted, furi-ous, distraught.

It takes a full week for the symptoms to even clear their throat preparatory to easing, a week I know that, once it is over, I will work quickly to put behind me, and forget, and start again. But while it lasts, it lasts forever.

Eventually, the conversation Jess had arranged comes around. It is to be me calling him, and as I dial, I wonder what to say, and how to say it. Hello, I understand you have fatigue? Hey! Me too! What's your star sign?

What if we have nothing to say to one another?

The first few moments are not unlike those on a blind date. He says hello, and I introduce myself. Well, I say. Yes, he says, and his laughter turns into a cough. I find myself wondering what he looks like, and also glad that I don't know. I tell him Jess said it might be useful for us to talk, or rather for *me* to talk to *him*. She has suggested that his improvements have been encourag-ing, and from this I will take encouragement myself. You might inspire me, I say, cheeks flushing. She has told me that he is back on his bike now, and cycles up to two hours a day. I say that it has been a long time since I cycled two hours a day.

I stop talking now, and wait for him to take over.

'Yes,' he says, 'it's true, I am making progress physically, but . . .' And here he stutters, and instinctively lowers his voice, as if imparting a secret. '. . . I've got to be honest with you here, mate. Emotionally, I'm coming apart. I don't think I've ever felt quite as bad as I do now, with home, girlfriend, work, everything.'

He goes on to tell me about it all, in detail, and I feel awful for him. I am hardly in a position to offer condolences, or support, but I try my best. I cannot quite work out whether it is the fall-out of the fatigue that has contributed to his emotional crash, but there is clearly a link, and it's one full of, for me, foreboding. I issue what I hope are not merely empty platitudes – I tell him how admiringly Jess has spoken about him, how brilliant his progress – and we part on good, friendly terms.

'If you ever want to talk again, just let me know,' he says, and then he laughs again. 'I'm not going anywhere.'

I put down the phone and stare at it, trying to imagine why Jess had thought he would be so useful for me to talk to. And I start to wonder whether what is happening to him is what lies in wait for me, too.

Work is impossible after this. I mull over the call and its potential ramifications, and feel ill. Already catatonic with tiredness, I am now freshly convinced that things will get even worse, and that I too won't be able to cope. I will let my family down, I will have to give up work in exchange for unemployment. And what will happen to me then, to all of us?

When Elena comes home, I manage, carelessly and with needless cruelty, to start an argument, to which she responds with shock, confusion and hurt. My accusations are weak, but I'm angry, and scared, I want to lash out, and I've nobody else to take it out on. We never normally argue in front of the children, and seeing their faces as they witness this up close is not a good moment for me. I go upstairs – I would have liked to storm up them, furiously, but can't, so trudge instead – and fling myself onto the bed in an explosion of snot and tears, all too aware of the ridiculous soap-opera moment I am creating, but unable to do anything, right now, to stem it.

After our next session, Jess concedes defeat, and refers me to her superior.

Meanwhile, London gets on with its business, and I can only sit at home and watch it on TV. Last year, it was the riots, which transformed the city in ways I had not seen before, and now it's the Olympics. A dozen of Elena's friends arrive from Spain, keen to soak up the atmosphere. They rent a house near us, and every day take the train into town, to the shops, the zoo, and over to the Olympic Park to mingle. My girls often go with them. I see them off in the morning, strapping their little backpacks to their backs, filled with snacks and water and suntan lotion.

'Come with us?' they ask.

They arrive home much later, exhausted but happy, their faces lit up with all the adventures of the day, both of them falling over the other to be the first to tell me all they have seen: the new stadia, the cheery volunteers, the friendly faces all round, the hotdogs they had bought and only half consumed, and the Cokes, too, in huge cups, 'and I finished it all, Daddy!'

I pull both to me, and hug them tight.

'You should have come with us,' they cry. 'It was fantastic!'

Nine

Jess's superior is a lady called Anna. I see from her photo online that she is pale-skinned, with bright, lively eyes and corkscrew curls. She explains in an email that it would work best to see me face to face, but I explain that this is not possible right now, so we agree to Skype.

But when the time comes, she calls to say that she is having a problem with Skype, so we must do our first session on the phone. 'Not ideal, but,' she says, and I can hear her shrugging. (The problem with Skype is mysteriously never rectified, and all our subsequent sessions remain via telephone.) Anna is one of the co-founders of the clinic, its Director of Psychology. She is a Cambridge graduate (albeit in linguistics) and, like Alex Howard, a former sufferer herself. She has a cool, crisp voice, alert and quick. If Jess resembled the primary school teacher she once was, Anna is more secondary school, and used to being in charge of wayward types who don't pay sufficient attention, the difficult ones. Her words are quick and precise, and she always sounds to me slightly impatient. I am aware every time I talk to her that everything she says is worth making a note of. It quickly becomes evident that Anna is good.

We begin. Anna talks about worry. The more we worry about something, she says, the longer the problem stays rooted in place. Worrying wastes energy, and I no longer have sufficient energy levels to be careless with. What I need to do now is explore how I feel about things in greater detail. I must work against the conviction I harbour that physical activity is in some way deleterious to me, because if I don't, I will remain drained, and train station platforms will extend tauntingly before me forever more. And we don't want that, she says. Instead, I need to reconnect with the belief I had before I got ill, that fatigue is merely temporary, and that the body is designed to recover. 'Stop being so over-protective of yourself,' she says. The less worried I am, the less anxious, the sooner I will become well.

This all sounds so simple to say, and makes such resounding sense. Then why, I wonder, am I finding it so difficult to achieve?

'We have a saying in the clinic,' she says. 'Your body isn't actually holding you back, it's holding you up.'

She goes on. All the functions that can abruptly flip into malfunction can be reversed. At the moment, my mind is working against my body; I need to get both working in harmony, in tandem. 'This is something millions of people around the world struggle with daily,' she says, a smile in her voice. The kindly assurance here is that I am not the only one. We all struggle to extricate ourselves from a variety of unhelpful responses. It is often difficult to correct them, but it is not impossible.

She asks me a question. 'If the fatigue you feel has an emotional contributor to it, what would it be?'

I am stumped. I understand each of the words separately, but together they don't seem to lead to an obvious answer. An emotional contributor, you say? 'Quite often, our emotional feelings can be expressed as pain,' she says, adding that she worries I may be thinking too much, trying to be too analytical. 'Stop with the analysis, and get more in touch with your emotions. Where are your emotions?'

She explains that my trouble is that I have now set up a whole raft of negative associations. Because I have had so much fatigue, I now anticipate it coming. It has become an irrevocable part of my life.

'But it has,' I say. 'That's unambiguous.'

'Yes, but there is a pendulum swing that exists between improvement and setback. So don't worry, because they are temporary ones. Over time, the good begins to outweigh the bad.'

Fatigue has triggered a strong anxiety within me. This, she suggests, is interesting, and surely pertinent. 'Can you think why?' she asks. I cannot, no. She suggests there is some kind of latent panic that has been lurking deep within my system, patiently, for years, possibly decades. It has now been suddenly set free. Why? 'Can you think of any panic or fear in your life, in your past?'

I think for a while, and come up with nothing. Anna is persistent. She wants to know about my upbringing, and I tell her about my single-parent family, my depressive mother, a younger brother who took their separation badly. 'And did you?' she asks. I say that after my father left, when I was 10, I was effectively promoted to co-parent. I think I did this willingly. It was required of me; my mother needed me. I loved my mother, but had never really got to know my father. He was always out, rarely at home, and when he was, he seemed tired, tetchy, quick to anger. He drank, there were arguments; a familiar story. I don't believe I ever really missed him. In some sense, I was glad he was gone. The arguments had stopped, after all.

Anna sounds relieved. I am at last talking.

'And how does this make you feel now?'

I shrug, before remembering to articulate the shrug for her benefit. 'Well, fine, I suppose,' I say. 'It was years ago. I dealt with it.'

'But not angry?'

'I don't think so, no.'

She sighs. 'Okay, try to imagine you are talking about somebody else now. If somebody else grew up in a similar environment to yours, single-parent family, mother depressed, a difficult relationship with a sibling, what kind of impact do you think that would have on the child? Would they feel safe, secure? Would they grow up, perhaps, with a lack of stability, a lack of the sense of solid ground?'

I must have experienced a sustained level of fear, she says, because what children need most in life is safety and security. 'Intrinsically, that kid would have to grow up with a lack of security, right?'

She asks me to imagine that child all grown up. What picture might we see? 'Basically, we learn the ways of coping in life when we are really young. If your way of coping with a lack of security as a child was to get everything right, to be as responsible as you possibly can, and then, in adulthood, to try to create a perfect life for your wife and your children, to not fall into the same trap as your parents, then this is the way you function in life.'

She says that once we set down a pattern like this, which we tend to do at around the age of seven, we keep playing that pattern throughout the rest of our lives, whether it is sustainable or not. The fear or anger I must have felt then hasn't gone away; I've just learned to squirrel it away. It wasn't sustainable then – I needed to stay strong for my mother – and so I don't have the vocabulary, or even the instinct, to verbalise it now.

People choose all sorts of ways to try to deal with their life situations and what they are exposed to. But this way of functioning may become unsustainable, and once there is too much pressure placed on the individual, then, over time, it might only take a trigger – an emotional blow, for example, a nasty virus – to come off the rails.

'Does this make sense?' she wonders.

She suggests that 'with this hypothetical person we are talking about, we know that there must be a level of insecurity at his core. He may well be a very functional person, even high functioning; someone who has grown up knowing just how to operate in the world. But there are landmines, something that can set off, or unlock, all that inner insecurity.'

She recommends I learn to understand what it is my body is trying to tell me. Something has come along to derail me, and in trying to get myself back on the rails, I panicked. Perhaps I am panicking now because I didn't after my parents' separation. Perhaps I am seeing emotional similarities between then and now. Was becoming ill and not recovering the trigger to send me into freefall, now terrified that my life would fall apart in a comparable way? That I would place undue pressure on my wife, my children?

'Does any of this resonate?' Anna asks me. 'Look, you can logically accept that this might be true, but I think there is a fair amount of resistance in you. Am I wrong? I sense a disconnection at an emotional level here.'

Because I have remained quiet, in fact silent, on my end of the line, she offers up a final analogy. If somebody is in a war zone, then while they are in it, they cannot really process what is going on. They cope because they have to. They do not develop post-traumatic stress until afterwards. We might be working with a similar pattern here, she says.

'What you remember from when you were a child is learning how to cope, and you had to because that was your environment. It sounds to me that what you did at that age was to disconnect from your emotional responses because they weren't helpful, and there was no space for them. You have to be strong and responsible. You have no opportunity to freak out, so you shut that away in a box. This is how we work, on an emotional level; it is what we do. We package things away, and get on with life.'

And so why, I ask her, when my life is steady and happy, is it all coming to the surface now?

'Precisely because you are so secure.'

I decide I have misheard her. Perhaps I phrased my question wrong. But, no.

'It's ironic, I know, but people tend only to manifest all this stuff when they feel safe enough to do so, at an unconscious level. The rule of the unconscious mind is that we will only release things at the surface of our consciousness, bring things through, at a point at which we are able to deal with them.'

'But I'm not dealing with them, am I?'

'I'm not suggesting this is exactly what is happening to you, and I could be wrong, but my instinct is that it has triggered something deep in you. You stepped on a landmine, and it exploded. It has probably always been there, this fear, but nicely packaged away. Not any more.'

I look at my watch. Time is up. She leaves me with an optimistic coda.

'You will have a lot more resources now than you did when you were seven, trust me. So you will be able to better deal with the issues. And it is all happening to you now so that you can deal with it now, so it won't come along and bite you in some other way in the future. A little part of you simply needs help, and is bringing this to your attention, literally. Remember, this is all very normal, very psychologically accepted. It is also entirely surmountable.'

It is around this time, and surely not coincidentally, that I find myself writing a newspaper article on the world of self-help books and the often self-appointed gurus behind them: who are these people, and why do they presume to have so many of the answers to life's more enduring anxieties?

I have never previously read self-help books, nor have I had any particular compunction to do so. I have browsed a few, but have always felt assaulted by the proliferation of exclamation marks, the goading bullet points, and the wearying proclivity towards indefatigable, and often nonsensical, optimism in the face of wretched adversity. For my piece, I speak to people for whom such books are bibles – 'They are my bibles!' one entrepreneur tells me, a woman who has read over 300 of them and is now running a mini empire as a purported result – and to others for whom they are not. 'I have never had any faith in any of that self-help shit,' says the offspring of one American giant of the genre, a man whose can-do books were global bestsellers for decades. As Dad was travelling the world imparting his family-centric motivational talks while having an affair with his masseuse, his son slid slowly but emphatically into heroin addiction, and later joined a death metal band whose canon includes songs with titles like 'Wrong Whole' and 'Pre-Emptive Priapism'. 'I guess I've always been drawn to playing really loud music,' he tells me. 'It's therapeutic, cathartic. And I needed the outlet, because I don't express anger all that well.'

A leading British novelist, meanwhile, who had read many self-help books for research purposes, tells me that 'so much of it is just a dreadful bag of charlatanry. *Every day in every way I am getting better*, they say. No you're not. You're dying. Every day you're getting closer to your grave.'

I reason that I may be more open to these books now that I am in a time of comparative need, and so I buy, and read, some of the most celebrated (and therefore pilloried) of them all: Dale Carnegie's *How to Win Friends and Influence People* (1936), Norman Vincent Peale's *The Power of Positive Thinking* (1953), M. Scott Peck's *The Road Less Travelled* (1978), and Susan Jeffers' *Feel the Fear and Do It Anyway* (1987). Each lecture on how to filter out the bad in favour of the good, how to take risks and run free, how to be, to breathe, to focus, not waver, not wallow, how to talk, and think, and listen, how to be good, how to love, and how to live in harmony, with spirituality or otherwise. The collective optimism on offer throughout these hundreds of pages is distilled into pure alcoholic potency that must speak terribly loudly to those who need direction, help, guidance. Each has been a totemic multi-million seller, and each has helped to spawn a genre that, by the early 21st century, has grown fat and bloated, and surely driven now by little more than cynical opportunism. We do not really need any more books with exclamation marks and bullet points essentially saying the same things only with different chapter titles, and yet still they come.

Over the next few months, many people I encounter will recommend titles like Rhonda Byrne's *The Secret* and Eckhart Tolle's *The Power of Now*, lavender-scented self-empowerment tomes with shiny covers and instruction on how to live life, but my instinct remains a reliably blind one: yes, all such titles may be full of good, solid, sound sense, but the way in which such wisdom is dispensed lends it all an air, to me at least, of parody.

And so I continue to find my literary sustenance elsewhere, with a steady diet of distinctly middle-aged memoirs that rhapsodise on decrepitude, illness, bereavement, misery and miserliness. Elena worries for me, convinced I should be reading happier books, but I argue that these *are* happy books, full of vivid life and bitter humour, and the most wonderful sense of optimism, albeit bruised and slightly dented. It's an age thing, I tell her.

Correspondingly, I begin increasingly to like music made by men with beards, and the jokes of comedians whose male pattern baldness gives them night sweats.

Anna continues to drill down into my upbringing, encouraging me to explore the hurt I must have felt over my parents' separation, and the role it foisted upon me, how sad it must have made me, how scared and angry. I can hear her frown when I tell her I always saw the end of their marriage as a purely positive thing.

We were at least able to start afresh. Single-parent-family status moved us to the top of the council waiting list, and within a year we had left the ninth floor of our block of flats in favour of a newbuild house, with a bedroom each and even a small back garden. This was progress. Then came a washing machine, a second-hand car, a cat. I enjoyed school, had friends. Within those boundaries, life, so I had always thought, was good. No?

'Can I point out the blindingly obvious to you?' Anna says, interrupting my reverie. 'You are now in a situation where you are out of control, losing your independence, where you are constantly frightened, and feel under threat. Does this remind you of anything? Your body is mimicking the exact situation you have been running away from all your life.'

I ask her what I should do about it.

'You don't need to do anything about it. Just start by realising it, by acknowledging it. Basically, say to yourself: Oh yes, shit, that makes sense. And repeat it until you get it.'

It seems that I have spent my life trying to protect myself from harm and hurt, from outside interference, from certain people and uncertain situations. This has left me with body armour that I have been lumbering around with, without my knowledge – until now.

'Our bodies are very, very intelligent,' says Anna. 'Suits of armour are heavy. They drag you down, make you tired.'

'But I don't need the armour any more, do I?'

'You're right, you don't. But there is a part of you that doesn't realise this yet.'

She says I should address my sub-personalities. 'Do not disown the words *protection, fear, armour*. Our unconscious mind works symbolically. And can I remind you that it was you who first mentioned having a suit of armour?'

She is right; I had. It just came out in response to one of her quickfire questions. I never even saw it coming.

'That's why it was in your subconscious mind, so trust it. I get it that it is confusing to you, and I don't for a moment feel frustrated with you, but what we have to do now is find a way to work with your very powerful mind and, slightly, try to get your mind out of the way. We are defined not by our rational minds, but by our subconscious ones. Okay?'

A few nights later, over a long post-dinner talk with Elena when we could have been watching television instead, she tries to shed light into my dim brain for me. I had been struggling with everything Anna had told me: its significance, and how to process it. Elena, all too evidently, has no such difficulty. She suggests that I am scared of being hurt because I have been hurt in the past. Even if I did not realise it, my parents' separation, and the subsequent fallout, put me in a situation where I needed to be, and remain, strong in order to survive, to put up parameters which to me felt safe, and in which I could operate, and live. I have been doing as much ever since. Whenever something looks like it could hurt me, I remove myself from that situation swiftly, body armour on, barriers up.

But then I became ill, and couldn't seem to recover. This was not part of my script, and so I panicked and had to realign the parameters. This is why I fairly quickly adapted to it, and learned how to survive in this new, compromised state. I could now exist at home, and be at least a present father to my daughters, and I could still work. For this I was grateful. But over everything else, I developed a heightened fear. I could not allow myself to be compromised further, and so I closed the door, both metaphorically and literally, in order to protect myself. Which is how I ended up stuck, which is why any activity outside those parameters left me flooded with anxiety and fatigue.

It is this, then, that I need to learn to manage.

'From a psychotherapeutic point of view,' Anna says later, 'the level at which you disconnected from your fears as a child is quite impressive. You did it very effectively. You parcelled it away so much so that it took really quite a lot to engage you with the fact of what is still there. You became ill, and something in you snapped. No longer could you override that fear. We need to now re-engage with that fear in order to work with it, to let it go. The disconnecting which you have done so well in the past is no longer working for you now. You have to stop disconnecting. You have to engage with it.'

Anna is happy, and I am relieved. We can move forward now. The next time we speak, she tells me we are in a process of recalibration. It might be slow, even dispiriting at times, and I will have to be patient with it, but I will get there. We speak once a week, then once every two weeks, an hour each time, then half an hour. When she tells me she is soon to go on maternity leave, I am in a way relieved. At first I had relied on our sessions, but as they progressed I had become increasingly aware that we were talking in circles, about the same things over and over again, and I no longer feel I need to hear it again. Her maternity leave offers a natural conclusion.

She suggests that a course in cognitive behavioural therapy might be useful. CBT teaches patients how to observe their thoughts and beliefs, and also how to develop the skills to influence subsequent mood and behaviour. When somebody falls into a negative pattern of belief, they can be taught to change their reaction to it, to lessen it, make it less harmful. It has proved very effective among people with fatigue, but also with depression, anxiety, phobias.

CBT is offered at the clinic, but at the usual fee, and I have long ago stopped being able to afford the clinic's fees. No matter, Anna says, because I will qualify to get the treatment on the NHS. Of this she sounds entirely confident. She wishes me well, and says: 'You tend not to recognise stress very well in yourself,

I don't think. You normalise it. You need to learn to recognise now when you are in stress, and also when you are in a healing state. It is being in a healing state that you have to maintain. That's the only glitch now, if you like. Otherwise, you are extraordinarily normal, and I hope you will be happy to hear that.'

'That's fine by me,' I tell her.

She says one last thing. 'I have never come across anyone who hasn't gone through what you are going through right now on their route to ultimate recovery. You would have to be Superman not to encounter stumbling blocks along the way, but, trust me, you will be able to cope with whatever you've got coming up.'

Though I don't know it yet, it turns out she's right.

Part Two

CURE . . . ?

Ten

We decide to go on holiday, Elena's say-so. She is convinced it will do me, us, good, our first holiday in two years, and a chance for me to travel further than the front gate, or the nearest Costa. Google estimates a five-hour car journey, but Google does not bank on a traffic accident just outside Paris, nor on the unexpected early death of Elena's iPhone battery, and with it the only satellite navigation system we have. This results in many wrong turns in what must be France's flattest, most unremarkable region. There are few signposts, and little to tell us where we are.

We arrive 11 hours after we had set off, all of us tired and exhausted, legitimately so. The owners have been sat in the garden with the keys waiting for us for hours, they say. Before they leave for Paris, they tell us that the small outdoor swimming pool is closed until August (it's June now), and that a storm is coming. Adieu.

The storm arrives within the hour, and the temperature plummets 10 degrees overnight. We wake up the morning after to find we really are in the middle of nowhere, but something inexplicable (to me) has occurred: for the first time in a long time, I awake without fatigue. It is as if, away from home, where I have built up such a store of bad memories, the maladaptive stress response has nothing to clutch onto, no negative connotations associated with the place. I still feel consciously fearful of overdoing it, but my subconscious knows better, and my anxiety loses its capital A. I wonder, only half-jokingly, whether it is possible to live on holiday, to never go home again.

When we return to London a week later, I make an appointment with the GP to request a referral to the local CBT clinic. The doctor looks from my notes to me with an unreadable expression on her face, asks me rote questions to which I offer my rote answers, and tells me that I shall be contacted in due course, 'to see whether you qualify'.

A few weeks later, the call comes. I speak with a lady called Phyllis, and we chat in a way that seems to me informal and friendly. At some point I say something that makes her laugh, a high, lucid giggle that is infectious. As we end the call, I find myself hoping that she will be my therapist.

Two weeks later, I receive a letter. It says that, regrettably, I do not qualify for CBT on the NHS. I call Phyllis to ask why, and she explains that I had not shown sufficient signs of depression during the initial consultation. Quantifiable levels of depression are required in order to qualify, she says.

Phyllis is apologetic and empathetic. In her opinion, she confides, she agrees that CBT would indeed benefit me, but she says that NHS guidelines are there to be adhered to. The questions she had asked me two weeks back are the same for everyone – it is a standard form – with not much room, she suggests, for individual expression.

Then she says something unexpected. How about we go through them again, now, and you reconsider your answers?

I am not sure what she is suggesting here, but it seems clear enough that I should answer them differently – in effect, make myself sound more distraught, less level-headed, and not even attempt to prompt that infectious giggle of hers.

A little bemused, I say okay.

Though I cannot quite confess to feeling suicidal, I do my best to tweak my answers accordingly, and try to convey what is an undeniable truth: I am unwell. I am miserable about it. I need help.

Our call ends, and she sounds optimistic. 'Great, thanks, I'll be in touch.'

She calls back a day later. Good news and bad, she says. Her boss still feels I do not fully qualify but agrees that certainly some sort of NHS-funded assistance is warranted in a case such as mine. What I do qualify for, then, is a few one-to-one self-help sessions with a counsellor, dispensed around CBT principles. But it is not to be confused with CBT, because it isn't, strictly speaking, CBT. It's more helping you to help yourself, through suggestion.

This isn't quite what I had requested, of course, and not what had been recommended to me by Anna, but it will have to do.

I thank her, with sincerity.

My first appointment is in three months' time. 'It's a long waiting list, sorry.'

The health clinic is a short bicycle ride from home. A short bike ride is something I can now manage, but not without a certain amount of mental preparation – and, if I'm honest, a helpless case of nerves that prompt an unhelpful spike in cortisol. My appointment is for 9.30 in the morning, and as I make my way there, my cloudy breath reminding me that winter is coming, I feel a mixture of excitement and trepidation.

It is a small, squat building located to the north of my neighbourhood, nearer the park, where there are Italian delicatessens, independent coffee shops and houses with bigger extensions. I am buzzed in, and walk upstairs to find two other people in the waiting room, a motorcycle courier in his 30s with Slavic cheekbones, and a young woman in her early 20s, her eyes shielded by a curtain of strawberry blonde hair. There is no eye contact between any of us, and I instinctively take the seat furthest away from either of them, next to an overgrown potted plant. I am given a pen and a form to fill in, which asks me whether I am depressed, suicidal, avoiding social situations. I chance a look up at the man and the woman, and realise they are answering the same questions themselves. As I find myself ticking No, I cannot help but wonder whether they might be ticking Yes.

Moments later, I am being led down a carpeted corridor by a woman whose official title here may or may not be 'caseworker'. She leads me to a corner room that hasn't seen redecoration in decades, and encourages me to sit. There are two low chairs arranged around an even lower coffee table, upon which is a box of tissues. I sit, and the woman smiles at me and tells me her name: Claire.

I recount my story, bored by now of my own words but at the same time invigorated, because I am hopeful that this time it may produce different results, that this new person opposite me – Claire, who is French, a few years younger than me, and radiating an almost maternal kindness (though I don't know it now, she is in the early stages of her first pregnancy) – might just be the person to make me well again. Her accent is ravishing.

She begins by telling me that I will be allotted between six and eight sessions, once a week, where we will discuss not so much my recovery as my attitude towards it. Because my condition is still so unchanging, so tedious in its repetitive nature, I readily accept the offer to talk to somebody about it. At home, I must be boring Elena senseless; the opportunity to bore somebody else holds much appeal.

However, I quickly become aware that this is not the form of treatment Anna had recommended at all, not even close. Though the sessions may be guided by the principles of CBT, Claire talks much more like the self-help books I recently read, albeit with less evangelism. In comparison with the sessions with Anna, the discussions I have here feel like a distinct step back, a waste of taxpayers' money. There is none of that forward-motion dynamism I had become used to at the clinic. Claire focuses on the management of my expectations. She says that what I am going through right now is a kind of post-traumatic stress, that the experience has changed my life completely, and so of course I am going to be anxious about it, and fearful. Who, in my situation, wouldn't be?

But there is hope, she says. She tells me that I do not present to her as other chronic fatigue cases (this may have been because I don't have actual chronic fatigue, though I still don't know that yet) and that this is to my benefit. She says that I speak with strength and conviction, that I walk from the waiting room to the consultation room quickly, often ahead of her. To her, I seem confident and capable. Her other patients, she says, are different. It is as if there is a cloud above them; you can almost see the fatigue. You can see they are depressed. Not so with me.

Each week we talk about the week before, the progress made in my thinking patterns, the need to focus on the positive and the improvements, and not the negative because the negative will only hold me back. About the frequency of the symptoms themselves, and the occasional gravity of them, she doesn't know what to say, nor why they are so persistent. She tells me to be positive, above all else be positive. It is all a bit comfort blanket, this, leaving me with a nice, warm feeling, but it is gentle, and gentle right now feels ineffectual and frustrating. I do not want to tread water, I want to plunge forward. After the sixth session, she asks if I would like to continue to eight, and I tell her no.

The last time I see her, shortly before she goes on maternity leave, she tells me that, all things considered, my life sounds pretty good.

'Things could be worse, you know?'

She is right, of course. They could. The noisy neighbour could still be living next door, but he isn't, he has sold up, and a much quieter couple have moved in. I could be bedbound, I could have lost my job, or else be as suicidal as the Q&A form I need to fill in each week persists in asking. But things could also be better. I could be well, walking again, running, swimming, cycling for longer than 10 minutes at a time. I could be shopping with my children, taking them to the park, the museum, anywhere. My aim here is to claw back some kind of normality. Is this too much to ask for?

If I am reading Claire correctly, then maybe it is, yes.

Right, so. A door has been slammed shut in my face. I have reached a kind of impasse, arrived at a dead end. Because I am not more seriously unwell, no concrete procedure available, that's it, I'm on my own. As far as the NHS is concerned, my life is already pretty good. Things could be worse.

But, no. I refuse because, frankly, I am not prepared to put up with the way things are now for ever. I have not acclimatised to my condition, not at all, and nor do I want to. I *want* to get better, to actively, proactively, become well again. I will not accept that this is too much to ask. From my nervy readings on the subject, I know that it is possible, entirely feasible in fact, and that if I do things the right way, it is realistically likely that I will not just improve but fully recover. Others have, so why not me? It is time to reclaim the world, or at least my small part in it.

The alternative – do nothing, put up and shut up – is not a viable option. I am not prepared for another three or four more decades of this. I have spent too long treading water. Enough. I have had enough. I sense that Elena has too, but she is too nice, too saintly patient (for now), to say.

I have had more than a passing thought of late that my condition might have done temporary wonders for our relationship.

Though we have always, I think, been strong, solid and still sufficiently happy with one another, we were nevertheless reaching the stage where, as newspapers like to tell us with irritating frequency, stagnation can and almost invariably does occur. That stagnation is why people have children, pets, and go into debt in order to have two weeks holiday a year. A change of dynamics, those newspaper articles tell us, and a change of scenery too, can perform wonders.

We had done all that. The pets, or rather pet, singular, was long gone, the children an ongoing project, and holidays were currently on hold. We were now mired in the daily drudgery of family life, and while this was enlivened by the routine thunderbolts of pure joy that only your children can conjure up, it was still a fact of life that our downtime now was comprised mostly of watching boxsets together, in companionable silence. Even a good boxset can only summon up so much excitement.

My becoming unexpectedly and, better yet, *enigmatically* ill, then, gave us something new to focus on, a novel pastime for the simple reason that it did pass time. Elena was brilliant: my carer, my nurse and educator. She continued to research the condition, and possible cures, at night, and often during days at work. Anything she suggested, I tried, and when I remained doggedly unwell, she was on hand to talk to, to sound off at, and to listen to me moan and grumble, pulling me as roughly as necessary from a trough of self-pity.

Evenings were now spent around the kitchen table essentially having the same conversation over and over again until we were both too tired to talk, while in the living room *Mad Men* remained unwatched. I marvelled at her patience, and then I worried over it, convinced it wasn't, and shouldn't be, finite. If my social life had unavoidably plummeted to nothing, it didn't seem fair that hers should too. I encouraged her to go out with friends, and she didn't need to be encouraged twice. When I bought her a few introductory lessons for salsa classes, she very quickly signed up for several more. She dressed up for it, with make-up. She looked pretty. It hurt to watch her go.

Though I have grown accustomed to solitude these past two years, I increasingly crave the company of other people. Anyone, I find, will do. One day, Jehovah's Witnesses stop by, two of them, male and female, both in late middle age, he the talky halitosis one, she with the vow of silence. I allow him to engage me for a full 20 minutes with warnings about the end of the world, which by all accounts is imminent, but not too imminent. 'It is foretold,' he says, pointing to a line in the leaflet that references Armageddon. He says he will leave the leaflet with me to read later at my leisure. We continue to talk at length now, shooting the biblical breeze, until he says something I thought no Jehovah's Witness would ever say: 'I'll let you go now.' And then he turns to go, still smiling his benevolent smile but striding down my garden path and onto the street, towards my neighbours. I very nearly follow him, wanting to cry out, 'No, wait! Come back! I've tea, biscuits!'

This is bad. Something has to be done. No, *I* have to do something. Me.

And so I do. I decide to write about it. In what form, I am not yet sure, but I will get it down on-screen, because if anything can help me to understand all this, and my progress through it, writing will. I am not sure yet if I will ever make it public, because my fatigue to date has been a strictly private matter, my business, my failing; I do not want to be judged by anyone else, and I do not want people to think that it has impacted on areas of my life that it hasn't. By which I mean work. I can still work. But writing about it could allow me to immerse myself in the subject from a constructive point of view. I could research it the way I would a news story, ideally well beyond its Wikipedia page. This might put me in an advantageous position because the more research I do, the more experts I might gain access to, experts I would otherwise never even know existed. And these people will be able to offer me a deeper understanding than I currently have into its cause and effect, the best ways to understand it better, to be less afraid of it and, perhaps, even ultimately to overcome it and leave it all behind.

Being a patient is to exist in a passive state; you become both noun and adjective. You sit there being given instruction by someone with greater knowledge, but the diagnosis is often brief and confusing. It all takes a while to settle, and the information can tip into overload, with only its headlines grasped. Sometimes you can forget much of what was said to you the moment you get back outside. Not the gist of it; the gist of it lingers like a bad smell. But the meat of it. Later, questions arise, not all of them hysterical ones, but there isn't always someone immediately available to answer those questions. And so they multiply, while others fall away. You find yourself wanting to go back in time to the initial diagnosis, on the promise that this time around you will pay greater attention. You might even take notes.

This is essentially what happened to me after I left Dr Dolittle. His vague diagnosis hit me like a thunderclap, but all I could remember afterwards was the thunderclap itself. I couldn't remember really what else he said, and for reference I had to consult with Elena because I had called her straight after my appointment, and she had retained what my mind had since so carelessly discarded.

Had I interviewed Dr Dolittle, on the other hand, emotion might not have intruded so much. I might have paid more attention and had the objective confidence to ask him more questions, some of which might have been penetrating ones that might have prompted illuminating answers. Most crucially, I would have recorded our conversation, which meant I would have been able to listen to it over and over again, as much as necessary.

The idea appealed, and motivated me. Of course it did; I was desperate, clutching at straws. But if nothing else, it would give me something to do. And it might just work.

Is it possible to write yourself better?

There are, I learn, approximately 465 alternative treatments out there aimed at people for whom mainstream medical advice has left them wanting. Presumably some of these treatments, many of them even, work? I will request interviews with leaders in their field, people with larger brains, better skills, greater knowledge. They can shed light on their work, my condition, and help me find a way out.

So if that door really has been slammed shut on me, maybe I can shoulder open another one and write up my experiences for my own benefit, yes, but also for others in similar situations in the hope that it might help them, too. I cannot be the only one behind a closed door.

This sounds like a plan.

Who first?

The offer of an interview with a motivational guru comes via email; his name I can no longer remember, and I would not repeat it here even if I did. Under normal circumstances, this email would have joined the dozens of other offers I receive on any given day in my Deleted Items, but I am immediately intrigued. His publicity people claim he might be the new Paul McKenna, the man who can make people sleep, thin, clever, happy. I look him up. Like McKenna, he is frequently employed in the world of big business and high finance, helping staff to focus themselves into being the best they can be, not just for their employers but also, presumably, for themselves. But he is good with phobias, too, and anxiety. One newspaper archly suggests he resembles Frank Spencer. I check out his website. He looks dynamic, his hair still redolent of the stylist's scissors, his teeth expensively dentisted. He boasts of his work with governments, how he always produces results and leaves people with a new zest for life. His promises are unabashed and boastful, his whole approach aggressively American. He can, he says, change your life.

Perfect, I think. I will interview him for a newspaper, then try to summon up the courage to broach my own issue on the side, and see where it leads. It is a prospect that unnerves me, though; I am not very good at this kind of thing. He is the subject, not me, and a journalist should never talk more than they listen, never take crass advantage.

I quickly hit what, in hindsight, is an obvious stumbling block: I cannot get my newspaper interested. No one really needs to read about a Paul McKenna-lite. It's a crowded area he inhabits, there are lots of him about, and there can seem something bullishly insincere about all of them. To many, they can appear opportunistic and ultimately vacuous, and no self-respecting editor would want to give very many of them the oxygen of publicity.

But I am desperate, and so I find myself emailing the man direct, almost against my will. I explain my predicament, my quest for knowledge, my aim to write about it somewhere, and I proffer myself as a viable case study. He has done bankers, MPs, all those arachnophobes, but can he heal the sick, someone with complicated sub-personality issues; me?

It takes him two weeks to respond. Come to my upcoming seminar, he writes, I'm sure we can work out a discount. I am heartened by his reply, and go online to read about it. The seminar focuses on honing in on one's managerial skills in pursuit of transforming a humdrum worker into a serious achiever, somebody worthy of promotion, a salary hike. We will leave the seminar newly invigorated and pumped up. We will have clear goals, and the tools with which to achieve them. The course is open to just 50 of us on a first-come first-served basis, so hurry. The charge is £500.

I email back to thank him, but explain that I am not the managerial type. Might he have any other seminars, perhaps more personal ones? Two weeks later, he emails back to say that no, he doesn't.

My plan has stumbled at its first hurdle. I write back thanking him all the same, and am surprised, a further week on, when he writes again. There is an alternative, he says. He sometimes works one to one, tailoring the sessions to the individual's needs. My excitement redoubles in an instant, and I look more kindly now at his picture on his website. I decide that he doesn't look like Frank Spencer at all, not really. The teeth, perhaps, a little. The tilt of his head. The beret.

I respond, and ask him to explain more, and he writes that, because of his busy schedule, we could work together over the course of a single day. We would meet in the morning and go on for as many hours as required. But I will leave cured. *Cured.* This is one of those words that the more you look at it, the stranger it seems. But it resonates on the screen of my BlackBerry, and I stare at it and stare at it, barely believing my luck. The lack of exclamation mark somehow makes his claim all the more powerful, because here is a man so confident in his abilities that he doesn't have to shout to get his message across.

'Interested?' is how he finishes his email.

Interested? Yes! Of course! I reply quickly, asking him to address the only thing he has failed to mention: his fee.

It takes a full day for his response to come. I count the seconds.

'£6000. Let me know.'

I email neurologists, brain specialists, and at least four pop and rock stars who have battled with fatigue but are, or appear to be, better now. The former and the latter never respond; the two brain specialists reply by saying they are too busy and cannot spare me the time. And then I encounter a friend of a friend who says he might be able to help. He suffered fatigue for several years. 'I tried everything,' he says. Nothing worked, but then he discovered that eating a whole clove of garlic each morning helped him get fully better. Perhaps I should try this myself, he suggests.

This comes close to defeating me: cure by garlic. It is a measure, I think, of a condition as vague and infuriatingly bespoke as this that vampire bait becomes a viable remedy. Little wonder it is so difficult for practitioners to agree on a single treatment, and little wonder too that so many find it hard to take quite as seriously as perhaps the condition demands.

At Elena's encouragement, I seek out a physiotherapist purely because, after two years of physical inactivity, I am bound to be stiff and inflexible. I find one who cites CFS in her past. She is based in a nearby gym.

At 17 years old, I read on her website, the physiotherapist sustained an injury that somehow led to irritable bowel syndrome and, by the age of 20, 'full-blown chronic fatigue'. Doctors referred her on endlessly, in the hope that somebody might be able to help. She eventually met with a cranial osteopath whose sessions she found powerfully altering. 'Many people noticed that I grew taller', she writes on her website. 'I found myself much less fatigued, lighter, and my digestion, skin and sleep, all improved.'

I book an appointment. In the flesh, she is tiny but wildly effusive, as if lit from within. I half expect to see a flex leading from her to a plug in the wall socket. She is all eyes and mouth and teeth, and she employs them simultaneously as she displays sympathy, empathy, understanding and encouragement as I tell her why I am here. She takes notes in the kind of handwriting only she will be able to discern – a long spidery scrawl – and interjects a lot, as if every time a thought dawns, she needs to air it immediately. She speaks without taking breaths, it seems. Great ribbons of words flow out of her; often I lose the thread. She says she has noticed that when I speak, my breath catches in my chest. This alters my voice, and denotes nerves, some under-lying anxiety. Not everybody would pick up on this, she says, but she does. 'I'm specially trained.'

On her website, on which she describes herself, disconcert-ingly, as a celebrity therapist for a prime-time BBC1 show, she speaks of her special techniques for sinus problems, dental issues, digestive and birth traumas. She also performs some-thing called fascial unwinding, a movement-based therapy used to unravel the body's connective tissue network which helps overcome injury and restrictions by increasing range of motion and function.

She asks me whether I believe I can get well, and I tell her yes, I hope so. But, often and more frequently, I do sometimes wonder whether I ever will.

'It's important you do believe,' she says. 'It's crucial.'

She puts down her pen and paper and says that she can help me, and that over the next few weeks – yes, she says quickly, almost impatiently, I must come back for more sessions – she will be asking me lots of personal, sometimes invasive, ques-tions, in order to find out more about me, and how I tick. Do I have a problem with that? The question is rhetorical, because she keeps talking. And, indeed, over the next few weeks, she will talk almost incessantly at me, proffering a great barrage of information both relevant and sometimes not. She tells me about her past, her many injuries and illnesses, the reaction of friends and family, her difficult boyfriends, some of whom were 'mad', one of whom had 'mad' parents. She tells me how one particular relationship problem was inadvertently initiated in B&Q when she overrode her partner's hunter/gatherer instincts by proving herself the dominant one when she lifted a heavy object in front of a member of staff. She boasts of her energy levels, which are constantly high, constantly firing, and of the zest she brings to the health club, which is what her colleagues always say, even those who don't know her very well. 'They say there is more energy about when I'm here than when I'm not!'

She tells me to lie down, and when she starts finally to massage me, it is unlike any massage experience I have had. She places a flat palm on my body, my chest, my arms, my thighs. In the expertise of her touch, she explains, its intrinsic know-how, energy will be brought up to circulate, released and relinquished. It will move where previously it had been blocked. As she does this, she asks me whether I feel any difference, any warmth or cold, and all the while she keeps talking, about her parents, her travels, about biology and science. Whenever a topic of conversation strays onto something negative – the recollection of an awkward moment, or else a painful one – she removes her hand to ensure that no negative energy is passed from her to me.

I leave my first session a little bewildered and bemused, but also sort of hooked. I have never met anyone quite like her. She is vivacious and serious, funny and smart. Most of what she tells me I almost immediately forget, but I conclude that it's my fault, my antenna faulty. Because her signal is clearly strong enough.

When I return the following week, she does more laying on of hands. The promised personal questions she mentioned the week previously never really come, and instead she tells me more about herself, events that have challenged her in some way, and she says that challenges are good, because what doesn't kill us makes us stronger, and that's the message here, the one to parcel up and take away, and unwrap in times of vulnerability. She strongly recommends I buy a particular medical book, one she had bought and pored over when studying to become a doctor (studies she didn't complete), and she shows it to me now, a huge, heavy, hardback thing, filled with hundreds of pages of colour diagrams of bones and veins and arteries, and expansive explanations on each, along with copious footnotes. It is not the kind of pop science book that makes it onto the front tables at Waterstones, not the kind of book I could ever read for pleasure.

By our fourth session, my confusion over what exactly may or may not be happening here is bleeding into nagging doubt. She tells me about extended trips to India, to yoga retreats, and she tells me about the former boyfriend she used to call Bilbo Baggins for reasons I fail to grasp, and as she talks and talks and talks, she places her fingertips, then her hands, and then her arms all the way up to the elbow on various parts of my prone body, and lets them rest there awhile. 'Do you feel the warmth?' she wonders.

Twelve sessions, she says, and then I shall start to feel some benefit. When I get home, I work out what 12 sessions will cost me. Elena asks if it is helping. 'Do you feel any better, any different?' The truth is that no, I don't. I am engaged by the woman, she fascinates me, and as life experiences go, this is undeniably a six, maybe even a seven, but I have little real understanding of what she is doing to me, or to what effect, and I am becoming impatient, too. There are, after all, approximately 464 other treatments I could be investigating. I might be wasting my time here when I could be spending my energies – a loaded word, these days – elsewhere.

Eleven

It is from a man called Ashok that I learn about something in the brain called the amygdala. It's tiny, located in the temporal lobe, there behind the ear, in the shape of an almond. It is most commonly associated with the fear response, and for those suffering chronically from fatigue, the thing is in perpetual overdrive. The American neuroscientist Joseph LeDoux has written extensively on the subject, and so it is him I contact for an interview. He responds with disarming immediacy, within a minute, declining my request.

According to LeDoux's writings, it is much easier to study fear than it is other emotions. As I have already learned, things that are bad have more impact on us than things that are good. He suggests that you can put such things as eating, drinking, even sex off for an indefinite amount of time, but fear you cannot. Fear you have to respond to immediately. The amygdala gets sensory information from the external world, from touch, taste and pain. When you encounter danger, you experience the fight-or-flight response and, thanks to the amygdala's efforts, blood pressure increases, the heart rate rises and stress hormones are released. It's a warning button, effectively, acting like that red cord in a public toilet all too carelessly pulled over and over again by people confusing it for a light switch, prompting baristas and train guards to come running.

But pull it too much and it doesn't retract, it remains over-stimulated and on a perpetual boil, forever convinced more

threat is imminent. By which time it has created Pavlovian association: we are forever on the lookout for the stimuli it considers
the most dangerous. And once we fall ill in this fashion, we
remain so.

What certain alternative practitioners strive to do when
attempting to treat chronic conditions is to quieten the amygdala, to teach the sufferer to metaphorically put an arm around
it, treat it like a friend, pop a cigarette in its mouth and tell it to
calm down, there's no danger here. Ashok Gupta is one such
practitioner. His programme is remote, accessed via DVD and
live weekly webinars.

Initially I consider contacting him for an interview, but I'm
having little luck in my interview requests, so instead pay the
fee and await my package. (I do eventually email him request-
ing an interview many months later, and he agrees. But the
day of our interview comes and goes without further word
from him.)

The package arrives on a Saturday morning. Amaya rushes
to receive it from the postman. She rips it open, and out
tumbles a DVD and CD boxset, alongside what looks like a
large poster folded up into a manageable square. I unfold it to
reveal a floor mat upon which read the words The Amygdala
Retraining Technique™.

'Amy-g. Dala,' Amaya reads, haltingly. 'What does it mean?'

It has a big circle on which to stand, and off it shoot arrows,
one red, the other green, one pointing towards Unwellness,
the other towards Health & Happiness. Along the latter are
further circles on which to stand, and that read, respectively:
Start, Breathe, Future Self, Reflect & Choose, Decision Making,
Visualise Health.

Evie joins her sister in looking confused. My self-consciousness ramps up.

'Work,' I say, folding it back up again.

I take the whole lot with me upstairs now to 'work', close the door behind me, sit at my desk, and begin.

The opening section features Gupta sitting doctorishly at his desk, a smile on his face. His thesis is that the amygdala plays a key role in the world of CFS. He quickly admits that we will find contrary evidence online (and I do), but explains that if we are going to follow his advice, we must do so fully, without the clutter and din of competing voices. Do not bother wasting your time with further visits to your GP, he suggests, 'unless they are particularly sympathetic. There is probably not a lot your doctor can do, in any case, unless you have other, secondary conditions which might require medical treatment.'

Because the amygdala's role is largely to decide when something is threatening us, and then to release an appropriate response in pursuit of protection, it is this, Gupta says, that we must focus on exclusively: controlling the amygdala itself. The brain can be rewired, reprogrammed. To do this, we need to stop all negative thoughts from filling up our brain, and instead lead it on another path, away from Unwellness and towards Health & Happiness. To do this, we must give the programme our unswerving focus, and prepare for an awful lot of repetition.

This is not therapy, he adds, but rather a process of retraining. This will allow me to feel in charge of my recovery and my training, because no one else can do it for me. "This can now be your responsibility," he says, pointing out that the word 'responsibility' comes from 'the ability to respond'.

Where the OHC asks for 90 days, Gupta demands six months. 'Make a commitment to yourself now,' he says, 'to give it 100% for six months.'

He wants us to embark upon a daily programme of work. This involves repeated viewings of the DVDs, and listening to the CD, and going over the accompanying booklet for greater clarity and, later, tuning into his weekly 90-minute webinars. These take place on a Wednesday evening, and in them he will develop his thesis and also update us on all the latest research. In turn, we will have the opportunity to pose questions the length of a tweet (typed into a box onscreen) which, if time permits, he will offer short answers to.

The six months sounds to me like a big investment, but the depth of his demand works in its favour. It makes you take it all the more seriously. That first impression I had of him – that here is a man I might trust – is compounded throughout my watching of the DVDs. And by trusting in his methods, I find I am starting to believe in myself. He clearly knows how to engender confidence in his work: he offers a full refund after six months to any of those who believe it hasn't helped.

The objective is to help us rewire our brain, to rid it of its recently developed bad habits. He says that what we have to do is fully tune into every thought, every half-thought the brain indulges in. Then interrupt it – more STOPS! – and think of something else instead.

'Imagine our mind is like a train that keeps chugging along. You have to interrupt its flow, its path. It should break that pattern of thinking completely. And if it doesn't? Simply do it again.'

The more we do this, he promises, the more our thoughts will be interrupted at a neural level, and therefore will create new neural paths, less anxious ones, more positive.

There is more. In addition to the incessant STOPS!, he recommends a daily morning practice: yoga, breathing exercises, a little meditation, then 10 minutes of powerful, healthy visualisation exercises. Recall a time when we felt truly happy, truly loved. Where were we? What were we feeling? Which colours would we associate with the experience?

Tune into it all as fully and expansively as you can, he says. Try to drum up a tingling sensation, goosebumps. Revel in the memory, call it up vividly, and stay with it for several minutes. Then repeat the exercise four more times, each time summoning up as much positivity as possible. Thrum with it, because the brain enjoys being in that nice place. It hasn't been in a nice place for a while now; it's time to reintroduce it.

Every practice needs a name, and so Gupta calls his The Hour of Power.

On the night before my first morning, I set the alarm clock for 6.50 a.m., entirely prepared for the fact that I will roll over and switch it off at 6.51, then sleep another hour. And yet, in the event, I awake earlier, impatient to get going. When trying to return to sleep fails, I get up, shower, do some yoga, some breathing exercises, my meditation, and run a selection of my life's greatest hits in my mind's eye. It all feels positive, proactive.

I do the same the morning after, and then the morning after that. Before I realise it, I have been doing it for weeks, weekends too. Occasionally I catch my reflection in the wall clock's face – not even seven o'clock in the morning and wide awake already, in the midst of a routine I would have scoffed at a year ago – and wonder: is this really me?

For the next six months and beyond, I maintain if not quite that same Christmas morning buzz, then certainly sufficient levels of enthusiasm to still get up and undergo a fairly lengthy stretch of methodical amygdala calming. In some sense, they are the best moments of my day: awake before anybody else, watching daylight creep across the early-morning sky, hearing my girls wake up, alert already, and racing across the hall to jump on our bed, only to notice me missing.

'Where's Daddy?' they ask Elena.

'Work.'

The yoga and meditation, at least for the time being, remain fairly minimal, no more than 10 minutes allotted to each, as per instruction, and if the breathing exercises are annoying – you have to close off one nostril with your fingers and breathe through the other, then swap, and I always somehow manage to smear a finger down the lens of my glasses – then at least they are brief, over and done with in five or six minutes. But it is the positive visualisations that offer the most fulfilment. It is not often on any given day you find yourself with time to conjure up, and revel in, some of your own personal highlights from life. I recall, in detail, time with Elena before the girls came along: Wengezi Junction on a sweltering morning in, truly, the middle of nowhere, wondering but not really caring whether the bus would ever arrive; dawn somewhere outside Mysore, the train tracks rattling beneath us, the holler of a tea wallah crying *chai! chai!* further down the overcrowded carriage, its sweet smell mingling with a hundred others, not all of them quite as sweet; waking up at Llulluchapampa campsite, almost 4000 metres above sea level, and taking in the exhilarating view of the clouds not above us but *below*; a small flat off Deptford High Street with too little furniture in it, where she took me into her bedroom for the first time.

And then the times with the four of us: cycling among thousands of others through the streets of a London closed off to all cars, ringing bells, honking horns and slaloming in and out of slowcoaches; wading through a waist-high, bath-warm Mediterranean Sea, one daughter tucked under each armpit as we looked out for jellyfish and pretended to be scared; and then, later, at night, the looks of delight on their faces when they realised that, yes, even way past their bedtime we were prepared to go out and buy them another ice cream.

It is on more than one occasion that the goosebumps are accompanied by a lump in the throat.

I go on to complete the six months, just as Gupta had encouraged. Then, aware that I am beginning to feel better than I have been for a long time, that my fatigue is becoming a different thing to me now, less fraught and more manageable, light at the end of the tunnel, I realise that I do not want to stop my morning's Hour of Power, and so I don't. Gradually, I begin to imagine myself doing this every morning now, a new, permanent routine, something I would previously have thought unimaginable, the holistic pursuit of somebody else, somebody wise, but not me.

I do not realise this at the time, but I suppose I am going through some kind of transformation here. Some people might describe it as a spiritual awakening, but I won't. Nevertheless, I have discovered something inside me I never knew I had, a something that has nothing to do with any sort of religion or higher power, but simply to do with *me*. It is me who has learned I have the power to affect my thinking, and for the better, to make me feel good, and happy, and motivated. The physical energy will return in time, but no more will I allow myself to feel quite so negative or despondent, or ruled by it, and quite so helpless. I like what all this is doing to me, how it is facilitating me, and freeing me up. No longer do I consider myself to be living under quite so heavy a burden, and I no longer consider my fatigue my own personal Incredible Hulk. These hours of power have allowed me to glimpse into my past – and the person I used to be, before illnesss – and they have helped me realise I can recreate that healthier mindset, and make it a part of my future, too.

Twelve

In the dozen years since my mother's death, I have made an extra effort to visit my grandparents in Milan as often as I can. I used to spend every school summer holiday there, when time for a teenager passed at a torturously slow pace, with nothing but MTV to alleviate my boredom. In my adult years, I have tried to visit at least twice a year, each a long weekend of pleasant inactivity, plenty of good food and the same old card games in front of the television. As an exercise in nostalgia distilled, it's a potent one: their home hasn't changed at all, and the same clock still ticks on the same mantelpiece, morning and night, chiming every quarter hour as if every quarter hour needed marking.

These times out from my life have never required much effort from me, merely a couple of cramped hours on a plane, a half-hour bus ride into the city centre, 20 minutes on a Tube, and a further 15 on foot to their apartment complex that flanks a busy road full of lorry stink, and finally three floors up to the small rented flat they have lived in for over half a century, and where they wait for me with open arms.

After my daughters were born these uncomplicated getaways became a little more convoluted, but following my grandfather's death, the visits took on greater emphasis, my grandmother now otherwise mostly alone. I did my best to increase my annual visits.

When the fatigue came, the visits shrank to zero. My every impulse told me to tell her, to explain, that she deserved to know why I was suddenly staying away. But when I conferred with a family friend, I was told, vehemently, that I shouldn't, absolutely not, that my grandmother would become sick with worry and fretting, and make herself ill as a result. My grandmother, she reminded me, was a worrier. But how to explain my abrupt absence, the fact that I was no longer visiting every few months? Every phone conversation we ever had had always finished with me saying see you soon, and her asking when. What would I say now?

For reasons I could never quite fathom – had the family friend said something, in some subtle way? – my grandmother never did respond with her routine 'When?' ever again. I had children now, and maybe she knew that that is what happens when you start a family: priorities, sacrifices. I felt dreadful about this, convinced she might believe I had forgotten her.

'Then let's go and visit her,' Elena says to me one night, plainly and reasonably, as if it were the simplest thing in the world. I look at her agog, and explain that if I still have difficulty taking the children to the playground, then negotiating an airport, a bus, its metro system and the long walk past the pet shop, the ice-cream parlour and the home-furnishing showroom en route to her flat was certainly too much. It is true that I am making progress, but I can't do this, not yet, I insist.

'Nonsense,' she says. She smiles. 'We'll drive. It'll be fun.'

It might also offer the two of us an opportunity for some extended time together, alone, something all parents not heading for divorce purportedly crave. We do. And I could perhaps use the opportunity to my advantage, to remind her that there is more to me, just, than perpetual sleep-hungry self-misery.

If my illness has brought me any real wisdom so far, as we are told illness is supposed to do, it is the knowledge that I married well. I had always known Elena was a strong woman, intelligent and passionate but also practical and seemingly unflappable. I have watched her bring to situations a sense of calm I would not have had a hope of bringing myself, and only infrequently would I wonder, when pricked, would she bleed?

But throughout this entire period, she has exceeded any expectations I may have had. I'm not sure how she does it. She tells me she copes because that is what people do when they have to. This is true, of course, but she has done so with a grace I would not have been able to summon up were the situation reversed. (It is only when I start to get better, incidentally, that she cracks and the pressure that has been building comes out.) My fatigue has affected her as much as it has me. Our lives have narrowed, plenty has been sacrificed, and we are both waiting impatiently for it to be over, to have finally evaporated and become a part of our shared history.

And so the idea of a road trip is exciting, on many levels. We have already lost ourselves, to a certain extent, within the mess of parenthood, and my condition has mostly cancelled out any lingering semblance of the people we had once been to each other. A road trip, then, will be good. It makes me nervous to consider it, but that in itself is no bad thing. Nervous is good; it is the precursor to adventure.

I like to think I had had a good relationship with my mother, someone with whom I could talk about most, if not quite all, things. With my grandparents, there was little we ever really said to each other outside the weather and work. How's the weather? Warm. And work? Busy. Good. Our unwritten familial law was never to burden one another with one another's problems; their directive, not mine, and one compounded by the fact that they couldn't speak English and my Italian was only falteringly fluent. When my grandfather fell at home and broke his leg, at the age of 94, I wasn't informed until he had spent almost a month in hospital. When I finally reached him on the phone, he insisted he was fine, and my grandmother corroborated the assertion, confident he would be home soon.

But he wasn't. He died in hospital while I was away for work. I missed the funeral. At the very moment they were cremating him, I was buying a new pair of trainers from a warehouse-sized shoe emporium that boasted considerable discounts. I spoke to my grandmother immediately after the service, standing on Wilshire Boulevard in the hazy sunshine, wondering why I was here, with my new purchase, and not there, with her.

Today, at 93, and now confined to an old people's home on the suburbs of Milan, my grandmother will still only ever admit to being 'fine'. She was forced to give up her flat because she was no longer able to live there alone, and needed round-the-clock care. But the transition from independence to assisted living discombobulated her. She sounded distressed on the phone, confused and angry. She could not hear me properly because she could not get her hearing aid to work; our phone calls often ended in tears.

Elena is right. We have to go.

There is a certain comedic element present in the undertaking of a road trip across Europe when I have grown accustomed to not travelling further than the garden path without keeling over in swooning exhaustion. And so en route sightseeing is out of the question because all I can do is look out the window and pine. Paris and its squirrelly arrondissements therefore pass us by completely. We miss the Eiffel Tower, the Latin Quarter and, worse still, we miss Shakespeare and Company, the best little bookshop in the world. While I sit in the passenger seat complaining about this, Elena reminds me that this is where we are right now, so let's just make the best of it, yes?

The whole venture requires careful planning. While I am prepared to undergo a necessarily restrictive, and very long, car journey with my wife, bringing the children along seems cruel. Keeping them cooped up in the back seat like unloved pets, with nothing but the promise of a care home at journey's end, is hardly Center Parcs. A two-week school holiday is looming, so Elena flies them to Spain to deposit them with their grand-mother, then flies back to me. The following morning, shortly before dawn, and too early to even attempt my Hour of Power, we are on our way. Elena drives, I'm shotgun, having long ago lost, or rather mislaid, my licence. I keep meaning to replace it but keep forgetting. We have no satnav, and so she expects me to be map reader. I gaze emptily out of the window.

Though she may suggest differently, we have always made for pretty good travelling companions, I think, a complementary yin and yang, as long as I get the aisle seat. She is the sensi-ble one, the one who books tickets ahead, does pre-departure research, books hotels and manages not to lose driving licences, while, to my mind, I am the freer spirit, happy to let the wind take me where it will – again, as long as I get the aisle seat. She has always wanted to plan holidays in advance, ideally secur-ing flights months before, while I am the more spontaneous, suggesting we go in a couple of days' time, whenever the mood takes us, and relying not on guidebooks but on whatever it is we possess that passes for instinct.

To drive across Europe now, however, Elena puts her foot down. She will be the one driving, so we need a plan. She wants to map out our route there and back, and for now shelves my suggestion that we drive home a different route in pursuit of a different view. She wants to book all hotels in advance, deciding upfront which towns we make our overnight stops in. I argue that we should just stop whenever it is late and we are tired. 'But you are *always* tired,' she shoots back, a little sharply. I try to suggest that an impetuous *Avez vous un chambre?* might be romantic. Yes, but where?, she insists. To this I have no answer.

All I know is that France is below us, and Italy below *it*. 'Just keep driving down,' is my advice.

Our first argument, consequently, occurs before we even make it to the outskirts of London. Our second takes place *quand nous sommes arrivés en France*, largely because I have started to respond to her increasingly impatient requests for directions exclusively in schoolboy French, thinking it amusing. This irritates her, but *je ne regret rien*.

We drive for hours in the direction of down, the motorways and their service stations eerily empty of other cars or their occupants. Where is everyone? It is just us out here, and the occasional HGV, no traffic, no roadworks, and nothing to look out at but an endless expanse of unremarkable fields that stretch to the horizon. I had no idea France was so empty or, for the car-trapped passenger, so dull. We stop for lunch in a small provincial town called Troyes, at the first restaurant we find. '*Un menu, s'il vous plaît*,' I ask. '*Menu? Non*,' comes the reply. The waiter points to every table in turn, each of which has on it the same big bowl of brown lentils and angry red saucisson, the house speciality. We order two. They arrive half an hour later, because why rush? It's Sunday. It is preposterously filling, the kind of meal that demands an après siesta rather than many more hours in the car. We are due at the care home within 48 hours, ideally, my grandmother expecting us. If she is wondering why we are driving across Europe rather than flying, and leaving the girls in Spain instead of bringing them with us, she makes no mention of it.

The journey continues dully. Elena suggests I sleep, but I cannot sleep sitting up, and I grow half mad with boredom (*ennui*) and clawing frustration (*frustré*) at this self-imposed incarceration, stuck in a Spanish-made hatchback that my wife is driving at the speed limit, and not a kilometre more, through a country in which all I really want to do is pull over, get out and wander around for days on end in pursuit of adventure.

'Shut up,' Elena says. 'Just shut up, and find out where we are on the map. Help a little, why don't you?'

It is getting late on our first day, and she has been driving, uncomplainingly, for hours, my saintly wife. We still do not have a hotel for the night, and the afterburn of the saucisson has lessened sufficiently for us to consider dinner.

'I told you we should have booked somewhere,' she complains.

Her fear is that we will be forced to sleep in the car, hungry, cold and cramped. I say that when we see signs for the next town, we leave the motorway, eat at the first restaurant we come across, then find a place to stay. *Non?*

Our third argument commences shortly after.

It does not happen much in our relationship that I am proved right and she wrong, but on this occasion it does. We arrive into a small, possibly nameless town, directly into its pretty main square. Here there is ample parking, and opposite is a restaurant, where we have *poulet et frites* with a bottle of pink *vin*, my first drop of alcohol in months. It tastes wonderful. A short stroll finds us a decent three-star hotel, whose well-appointed room we make use of in the way we would have back in the early days of our courtship, and we awake the morning after to sunlight streaming in through the windows, both of us exhausted, but in the very best way.

The following evening, another great swatch of featureless France covered and now mercifully behind us, we pass through the Alps and into Italy. The difference is as stark as it is abrupt. Suddenly, there are vehicles everywhere, a carnival of tooting-horn chaos as careening trucks compete alongside ancient Fiat 500s that are driven too fast by fat men asleep at the wheel. For the first time in our trip, I have to faithfully fulfil my co-pilot duties, sitting up straight, turning the music – John Grant's *Pale Green Ghosts* – off, now all eyes and ears, instinctively slamming my foot to the floor whenever another truck lurches into our path and prompting me to shout STOP!, STOP!, STOP!, thus no doubt confusing my neural pathways but helping Elena to keep us alive and avoid what otherwise seems an inevitable head-on collision.

We finally pull up, comprehensively rattled, at a pizza restaurant, where we talk about our daughters' lack of godparents, and whom we would appoint as adoptive parents if, as now seems quite likely, we do not make it to Milan alive.

This leads to our fourth argument, which, after a cold night in a bleak motorway hotel and over a continental breakfast the morning after, becomes our fifth.

The outer suburbs of Milan are about as easy on the eye as the outer suburbs of Nottingham or Walsall. It is propulsively over-industrialised, its roads flanked by factories, its high-bricked walls liberally graffitied with the very best Anglo-Saxon swear words, and all of it a world away from the Italy of tourist brochures. When we arrive, it is raining.

But there is relief to be out of the car after two solid days of driving, and we are glad to be here. The care home's design will win it no architectural awards, but it is clean and basic and functional. That it is my grandmother's home now, and probably will be for the rest of her life, is an abruptly sad realisation. I miss the flat she had shared with my grandfather for much of their lives together, and my times with them there. Never again will she make me lunch; never again will we sit around the dining table playing cards.

We find her upstairs in the cavernous, light-filled dayroom, where she looks wan and misplaced. Our reunion, as witnessed by two dozed fellow residents, is a muted one, none of the usual fussing, but for this I blame the new environment and the alienation she feels within it. We leave the dayroom for her room at the end of a long corridor, which she shares with a woman even older than she is. When we enter, the woman appears to be in distress, or perhaps it's pain. She moans in a low, steady voice. My grandmother, normally keenly aware of the suffering of others and always ready to help, ignores her. Instead, she retrieves a packet of biscuits from her bedside table and offers us some. I don't know how to interact with her here, everything feels out of place, and she isn't talking to me, either. Instead, we leaf through old photograph albums in silence as I desperately think how I can possibly alleviate her wretched situation and conclude, bitterly, that I can't.

We spend just two days with her, sitting in companionable, if always awkward, silence. She seems adrift, as far away as I have ever known her. The only time she really talks is to communicate her anger at being here, the cruel theft of the life she knew and her independence. (Within six months, we will, with the help of friends, have moved her to another care home outside the city, and here she will begin the slow process of acclimatisation and acceptance.) One afternoon, we leave the compound for a small outing, a walk, which I imagine is as much a novelty for her as it is for me, though I cannot of course communicate this to her. I am sure that my amygdala is firing its central cylinders, and that, under normal circumstances, I would be doing my level best to douse its fire, but right now my focus is solely on my grandmother. This helps. She grips hold of my arm with a tenacity she has brought to so much of her life, and we walk alongside one another, her surely holding me up as much as I am her.

At one point she looks up at me and smiles, maybe in nothing more than relief, and for a moment I feel capable, strong, if not in myself, then at least for her. Almost immediately I recognise it for the unusual sensation it is, me offering strength for someone when strength is what I have been so lacking of late. And in this instant I am not only glad that I came, but relieved, too. My grandmother needed me, and despite everything, I was able to come to her.

The journey home is gruelling, and more boring still, though Switzerland, my favoured route back, proves prettier than France, and the chocolate on sale at the motorway service stations of superior quality. We miss our allotted Channel Tunnel train by a cruel 60 seconds, and the two hours we are required to wait until the next one do not pass in a flash. I sit down somewhere, while Elena queues for duty-free wine. We arrive home late, and tired, and rise the next morning early in order to cross London again, this time to Stansted to meet our girls.

I had made this journey myself many times in the past, crossing town to greet my family coming back from Spain, butterflies in my stomach in anticipation of seeing their faces before they saw mine, these two beautiful, perfect little girls – mine, somehow – dressed in new clothes and sporting new haircuts, at once different and yet so very familiar. I would stand there alongside everybody else at the customs exit, waiting for the moment – and enjoying every drawn-out second of it – until our eyes eventually met and then, carelessly abandoning their Trunkis, they would run up to me, crying out 'Daddy!', while I dropped to my knees to scoop them up.

I have not been able to do this for what feels like a long time now, and I have missed it. So I am excited, and feel grateful, to be finally here, now, again. Elena has mostly recovered from our European trip, her body enviably good at revival, but my fatigue is powerful and all-encompassing. It will leave me feeling dreadful for weeks.

But it is worth it. Going on an adventure with my wife again, seeing my grandmother again, being at the gate to collect my children again: it is worth it.

Thirteen

One afternoon, a few months after Italy, I drift towards the bowels of my local bookshop, where the footfall is sparse and the carpet thicker, self-consciously browsing the self-help section. The name Eckhart Tolle has been mentioned again to me as the alternative health guru of the moment. His book *The Power of Now* is a modern-day Bible, it seems, always in print, always selling, equally adored and mocked, the true measure of success. Tolle is a German with complicated facial hair who lives in Canada and who spent much of his life, he explains in the introduction, in a suicidal depression. But then he underwent an 'inner transformation' and suddenly found that the world was in fact a miraculous place, 'and deeply peaceful, even the traffic'. It was on a park bench in London's Russell Square that he found this state of deep bliss, then he went away, replaced the bench for a desk and wrote *The Power of Now*, his guide to spiritual enlightenment in which he discusses, at length, the importance of living only in the here and now.

I leaf through the book for a while, but my attention won't focus, my resistance to these sorts of titles stubborn, so I put it down and walk over instead to the Smart Thinking section. I have only rarely strayed here in the past, always half-convinced I might be asked to leave, but I come across a book that catches my eye, and that appeals more than Tolle's. It is called *The Brain That Changes Itself: Stories of Personal Triumph from the Frontiers of Brain Science*, by an American doctor called Norman Doidge, and it recounts stories of people whose brains have been damaged in a variety of ways, through injury and illness. These include the 89-year-old who reversed his memory loss within six weeks; the stroke victims who learned to move and talk again; the woman with half a brain that rewired itself in order to compensate for the half it lacked. The book's central tenet is that the brain is plastic and malleable in ways we had never previously fully realised. On the flyleaf, neurologist Oliver Sacks gives it high praise: 'A remarkable and hopeful portrait of the endless adaptability of the human brain.'

It is part of a buy-one-get-one-half-price deal. I buy it. It's fascinating. I read about the woman building herself a better brain, about neural stem cell rejuvenation, and how one can use the brain's plasticity to help ease, even quell, worry, obsession, compulsion and bad habits. It is this bit that interests me most, and though this particular chapter focuses more on acute obsessions and compulsions, I recognise some of me in its pages.

'We can all experience such thoughts fleetingly,' Doidge writes, explaining that anyone can fall into destructive brain patterns, and that a great many of us do. Those who are trapped for too long, whose brains do not move on, begin to suffer, and do so in all sorts of ways. But the suffering is reversible. If the brain is plastic, plastic can remould. It can change. What we learn can be unlearned, because the brain needs never stop developing and correcting its mistakes.

I like the way Norman Doidge writes, and so I contact him for an interview. His assistant declines my request, *plus ça change*, so I turn back to the book. He writes about meditation and its myriad benefits. The more we are able to take a step back and observe our issues rather than engage in them quite so obsessively, he suggests, the more we can separate ourselves from them. And we need to separate ourselves from such issues if we want them to diminish. Meditating can help us teach our brains new skills, and the more we readapt them, the more they can be rewired.

I have been meditating for almost a year now, but it always feels half-hearted, a little too DIY. I approach it with ignorance, and sometimes impatience. But it no longer feels enough to simply sit on my office chair with my eyes closed for a few minutes a day, and so I decide, now, late as I am to everything in life, to do it seriously, and properly.

A few months previously, Claire, the NHS self-help practitioner who was not permitted to teach me CBT skills due to my insufficient suicidal urges, encouraged me to look into mindfulness, convinced it would help. She did warn, however, that I might struggle, and might not be able to sit still for more than a few minutes at a time, advice that struck me as not particularly helpful.

'You and I are alike, I think,' she had said, smiling gently, explaining that she had recently graduated from an eight-week mindfulness course herself. 'I found it very difficult at first, so do be prepared.'

I took offence, of course, and thought to myself: how dare she? The woman barely knew me. It was only later that I wondered whether she might have been doing some of that Waterstones's Smart Thinking on me, waving a red flag before what she knew was a very competitive bull, and thereby all but guaranteeing I would subsequently apply myself to the task more strenuously than I otherwise might, if only to prove my own private doubts wrong.

When I first considered learning to meditate this time last year, the practice still seemed stuck in the '70s, and was viewed accordingly. But something curious has happened over the last 12 months. Suddenly mindfulness is everywhere, and everybody seems to be doing it, many proclaiming remarkable results. In another year, it will have reached saturation point, and the newspapers will be full of stories of potentially harmful side effects (the result, largely, of endless self-appointed practitioners who don't really know what they are doing, or how best to train people in it), but right now it is the thing to do, and then recommend to your friends.

The man partly responsible for its initially quiet, now emphatic, rise is Professor Mark Williams, a clinical psychologist who worked at Oxford University and whose research centred around the treatment of depression. He appears to be the quintessential Oxford don, learned and studious, and nothing at all like a guru. But mindfulness actually originated in the United States several decades previously, the brainchild of one Jon Kabat-Zinn. He was a professor of medicine at the University of Massachusetts Medical School who developed it as part of a stress reduction programme. In its essence, mindfulness is 'the quality or state of being conscious and aware of something'. It is about focusing not on what happened yesterday or tomorrow, in half an hour's time or later tonight, but rather – much as Eckhart Tolle espouses – on what is happening now. It is about accepting your feelings, and your thoughts, and your bodily sensations, and how when you take a step back from something, you get to view it dispassionately, objectively, not subjectively. Everything can change as a consequence. So, when you drink a cup of coffee, don't just drink it, but feel the cup in your hand, its handle, the sensation of your lips on the rim, the drink itself on your tongue, in your mouth, your throat, its journey towards your stomach. As it is being served, notice your barista. Is she Polish or Czech? Eye colour? And now feel the chair you are sitting on, its fabric, the position of your elbows on the armrests, your feet on the floor. What about outside? Is the sun shining? Are the clouds cirrus or nimbus? What time is it, the hour, the minute, the second? How many carrier bags is she carrying? What did he just say? And so on and so on, extrapolated to all areas of your life that are happening in the present tense, the now.

I am beginning to see what Claire had meant: this will be hard.

Professor Williams is a skilled guide, though, and his meditations require neither Muzak nor sound effects, nor even an exaggerated voice that strives for equanimity by softening the consonants and elongating the vowels. Instead, he speaks normally. But then he does have the advantage of a wonderfully soothing voice. He sounds like an Open University lecturer, everything slow and effortlessly modulated, the Queen's English as it used to be before the 21st century arrived to ruin everything. I can tell he has a beard before Google confirms it; he probably has elbow patches on the jackets he wears.

'Each breath is unique,' he intones in the meditation I access free via Spotify. (Spotify clearly doesn't know quite how to classify him. Related artists, according to the site, include Dame Shirley Bassey and Martine McCutcheon.) Williams has a variety of meditations available here, their only real difference being length, one 10 minutes, the next 20, the final 40. Convinced I have something to prove, I plump for the 40.

Sympathetically aware that by three minutes in, some of us might be losing the will to continue, he readily concedes that our minds might well have wandered, because this is what minds do. When this happens, we simply bring our focus back again, as often as necessary.

I somehow survive the 40 minutes, and it feels like an accomplishment. Before I know it, I am doing two sessions a day, 80 minutes of sitting still. I do not find the meditation particularly easy, as Claire had predicted, but something about it feels right, and good. Every time I do it again, I am glad to have done so. Nevertheless, I am aware of a certain Achiever Type pattern running here: I am meditating because I have been told it is good to meditate. Therefore, the more I meditate the more likely it will be I get better, and quicker.

The trouble for me is that my mind never does fully settle, and there is always so much going on up there that I become increasingly convinced I'm doing it all wrong, and that it could be having little or no effect.

After one session, I make a note of all the things I remember had crossed my mind during it, and even as I write them up, I am confident I must have forgotten at least 70 per cent of my pointless wanderings. I thought about my children, and looked forward to when they would be home. I found myself rewriting an earlier email to an editor, then about rewriting the rewrite, and so I did so, word for word. 'Best', or 'Best wishes' at the end? 'All best'? I mentally tweaked the opening paragraph of an article I was writing about a TV programme, then drifted off to think about another, *Boardwalk Empire*, a new series of which was starting soon. And then everything else came in a messy, vaguely connected synaptic rush. Steve Buscemi, Graves' disease. Chocolate, coffee. How many pages left of the book I'm currently reading, and what will I read next? The fridge, how empty the fridge is. Need to stock up. *Sometimes the mind wanders for a little while, sometimes for a long while.* I'll buy more noodles. I like noodles. Soy sauce. Now I am thinking about Japan, Tokyo to Osaka, the bullet train, and the way the ticket inspectors, white gloves on feminine hands, bow from the waist as they enter and exit each carriage. So polite. That email again. 'All best, Nick.' *And using these stretches of silence to carry on the work by yourself.*

I try to focus on the breath, the sounds from outside, the birds, the buses, the postman. But then I'm thinking about a specific postman, the profoundly deaf one who doesn't know his own strength and who hammers on our door first thing in the morning, waking us with a terrible fright.

And on and on it goes, one errant thought bleeding into the next and the one after that, an endless swirling carousel, my brain incapable of any kind of focus, much less of stillness for peace.

I failed all my exams at school the first time around. This had surprised me then. It doesn't now.

The nagging sensation that I might be doing it wrong prompts me to contact an expert in the subject, Dr Danny Penman, who co-authored with Williams *Mindfulness: A Practical Guide to Finding Peace in a Frantic World*, a book that is on its way to becoming a modern bookshelf staple. It has sold a million copies since its publication in 2010, and has been translated into 30 languages.

Dr Penman speaks to me about stress, how everything boils down to stress in the end, whether we are conscious of it or not. 'Meditation is all about easing anxiety and stress,' he says. 'It manifests itself in everybody in different ways, but it's all linked, ultimately. Anxiety, cold sweats, panic attacks, depression, insomnia, exhaustion, fatigue – it all points to a disturbed mind, a disturbed way of approaching the world. Put too much pressure on it, and you begin to crack in so many different ways. What mindfulness is fantastic for is putting things into context, and in doing so, reducing that stress.'

He tells me that if we manage to remove the stress we are feeling, then our body will speed up the process of healing and revert back to its optimal state. Stress simply retards the optimal state and helps keep us ill, sick, chronic. Meditation can be used not just to calm the mind, but is also great for other things, like pain relief.

Mindfulness, he tells me, is all about acceptance. 'Accept your flaws. Not in a fluffy, self-indulgent, wallowing-in-your-own-problems kind of way, but just accept that you are human, that you suffer like everybody else, and that sometimes life is good and sometimes it's bad. That's just the way things are. Acceptance of the situation you are in is hugely important.'

This is something I have not done yet.

I ask him if it is possible to do meditation wrong.

He smiles. 'You are not doing it wrong if you approach it in the right spirit. If the mind is constantly hopping around, then don't worry. It's what our minds were designed to do: to collect information. So that's quite normal. The fact that you notice your thinking, and begin to notice the thought process itself – *that* is the meditation. That flicker, that moment of awareness: that's meditation. You are consciously aware of thoughts bubbling up, observing them, not being lost in them. This is where the benefits of meditation occur.'

It is the nature of the human mind to race and gallop along, he says. 'If somebody tells you not to think of a white bear, under no circumstances think of a white bear, then you will immediately start thinking of a white bear: why is it there, what is its significance? Instead, just observe each thought as it arises, then allow it to drift past your consciousness. Your mind will naturally begin to still, and benefits will gradually accrue.'

I interject here. I want to know about the *gradually* bit. How long, I ask, until you become aware of the benefits?

'Over time, your mind will become less fevered,' he replies. 'Your stress levels will begin to decline, and your body will begin to repair itself more efficiently. You will become healthier.'

Yes, but—

'Don't intellectualise. Just let it happen.'

I ask whether it is necessary that meditation be painful. I have read that many people choose to go to ashrams and spend 10 days kneeling on a hard floor in search of inner peace, often enduring considerable discomfort along the way. I tell him I sit on an Aeron chair, in tilt mode. Is that okay?

I am reassured by his answer. 'People in the East kneel or squat because that is how they have sat for centuries. For them, it's comfortable. In the West, we tend to sit on chairs. So if you want to sit, or lie down, fine. Just don't fall asleep. It's far more important to be relaxed while meditating than to be in any kind of discomfort.'

Finally, I ask whether he has ever found it boring, this tauntingly slow process of sitting still, doing nothing, while life races on around you, without you.

He laughs. 'Well, I'd argue that it's no more boring than brushing your teeth. I wouldn't necessarily suggest meditation is something you actively enjoy, it's more something you do because of the benefits it brings, and the clarity of thought. So if you are a little bored, that's fine. Just stick with it.'

In his book *Get Some Headspace: 10 Minutes Can Make All the Difference*, Andy Puddicombe writes: 'This is meditation, but not as you know it. There's no chanting, no sitting cross-legged, no need for any particular beliefs . . . and definitely no gurus.'

If the current craze for mindfulness has a poster boy, then it is almost certainly Andy Puddicombe. He is a fortysomething former monk and, he claims, circus trainer, a handsome man who boasts fine bone structure and an Abercrombie & Fitch dress sense, and is always photographed smiling widely. Do Headspace and you can smile too, seems to be the suggestion. The *New York Times* has said he is 'doing for meditation what Jamie Oliver has done for food', a quote money can't buy, and this has helped his book become a global bestseller, as well as its accompanying app sensation that now allows everybody to meditate on the go. Headspace was launched in 2010. At the time of writing, it boasts well over a million subscribers.

A friend introduces me to Headspace, approximately six months before Puddicombe starts to become the toast of the broadsheets, in which profiles on him claim his company is now worth somewhere in the region of £25 million. No wonder he smiles so much.

The Headspace website, with its bright colours and pretty layout, is appealing. It has something inclusive about it that makes each new visitor feel like a member of its special club. While you sit before your PC or tablet in preparation to meditate, for example, a little box onscreen tells you how many people are also using it alongside you. The first time I do it, at 1.30 on a Wednesday afternoon, 1,873 people have also set their sandwiches aside in favour of a little quiet time. A year later, that figure will be over 10,000.

Puddicombe himself is the guide, and he sounds pretty much the way he looks, and he looks very can-do, the kind of man who knows how to put up a garden shed without fuss. You trust him. He tells you to close your eyes, to breathe deeply, to count your breaths. And that's it. At the end of the 10 minutes, he is genial, matey. 'So, how was it?' he asks.

It's very good. I do it for several weeks, then several more. I contact Dr David Cox, then (but no longer) Headspace's chief medical officer, for more information. I ask him about the sudden rise of mindfulness, and he tells me there is little mystery to it.

'It is the right antidote at the right time,' he says. 'Everybody these days is talking about society being affected by hyper connectedness, 24/7 working patterns, social media, people being addicted to their phones. And the scientific community is beginning to realise that this is having very specific effects on people, particularly in the Western world. We have developed a reduced attention span, a reduced ability to focus. There are various emotional impacts that come from this.'

Cox is a former NHS doctor who quit after the stress of the job was compounded by the fallout from his father's death. 'Things were starting to get pretty heavy,' he says, 'which led to me starting to look for different ways to deal with all this stuff.' He developed an interest in mental health, and came across Puddicombe's work. Puddicombe was himself keen to bolster the credibility of meditation within the modern world, and promptly employed Cox as chief medical officer. Since leaving that job, Cox has become involved in academic research and finding convenient ways in which meditation can be implemented into the workplace.

He tells me that we have lost our ability to disconnect, to fully take time out for ourselves. We are fearful of switching off, of missing out (within a year of us talking the acronym FOMO – fear of missing out – will have made it into the *Oxford English Dictionary*), and we need to be constantly updated irrespective of how much this might drain us.

'Evolution is a wonderful thing, of course, and we will adapt, but we've been around for 100,000 years or so, and evolution happens on a very slow timescale. But what's happening to our society now is happening very quickly. It's 200 years since the Industrial Revolution, and our brains are struggling to cope with the way we are living our lives now. Yes, we have it easier than people had it before, in terms of ease of access to shelter, to safety, to food, but we are being bombarded with information in many different ways, at incredible speeds. We have never experienced this before, and our brains are struggling to cope.'

There are some who might challenge this, rubbish it even. Not all of us, after all, fall ill because of our smartphones, our tablets, and not all of us register such a severe depletion of energy simply because we are *on* all the time. But Dr Cox insists that it does deplete us all, every one of us. It wears us down, and affects us in all sorts of ways, whether we realise it or not. 'And this is why we increasingly hear from so many people who say it takes some kind of physical or psychological shock to occur before they start to look outside their normal boundaries and do something to help themselves.'

A recent Harvard study revealed that the average adult spends 47 per cent of their waking hours with their attention not on what they are doing, but elsewhere. This means that almost half our lives pass us by while we are lost in thought, worrying about the past, fretting over things that haven't happened yet.

'The whole concept of being in the present moment, having your attention in the here and now, is an interesting one,' Cox tells me. 'Our psychology is designed to scan into the future and look for possible danger. When anything has happened, we access our memory banks and look into the past to see whether we have ever been in a similar situation. What happened then? What was the outcome? That was a very powerful tool, and still is, evolutionarily speaking, but what it means is that we don't spend a lot of our time paying attention to the here and now.'

The point of mindfulness, says Cox, 'is to take that little step back and not get quite so emotionally bound up in thought'.

This is why mindfulness has proved so successful in dealing with depression.

'It doesn't necessarily change your thinking,' says Cox, 'and we're not trying to take away that evolutionary impulse. But what mindfulness does is to give you a healthy distance from those negative thoughts so that you can be aware of them, you can watch what is happening. You learn to recognise when your thoughts have raced off into the future and you are busy catastrophising about something awful that might happen next week. Psychologists have a wonderful term: cognitive fusion. This means that you are absolutely bound up in the emotional content of your thoughts. You perceive them to be absolutely true, you are emotionally fused with that thought. Mindfulness teaches cognitive *diffusion*, the ability to take that little step back, and not be quite so emotionally bound up. This doesn't mean we no longer have emotions, and you don't experience anything less in the moment; it just means that you are able to appreciate what is going on internally as well as externally. You are never going to stop your mind from wandering off, and you don't want to. You just want to learn to be aware of when it does.'

Mindfulness is not about entering into a trance state, he adds, which is good because not all of us have the focus of Buddhist monks.

'Whether you reach a kind of trance state is not the goal here. Clearly many people do, but that's not what we're aiming for. It's also not necessarily where you derive the most bene-fits from.'

I ask whether it is possible to do meditation wrong.

'No. You are almost certainly doing it right. Why? Simply because you are trying to. It's a slightly elusive thing, though. When you get it right, you don't all of a sudden enter into another state of mind. You are simply trying to pay attention to the here and now.'

This all sounds good and encouraging, I say, but there are so many competing meditation practices out there. Which is the best? Which should I choose?

'You know you are doing the right one when you try it, you like it, and you keep doing it,' he says.

I do it every mid-morning, or else early afternoon. I never miss a day. I visit the website, check to see how many other people are doing it with me, and let Andy Puddicombe talk me gently into mindfulness. Afterwards, not immediately afterwards, of course, but afterwards in the sense that, post-meditation, my senses are freshly alert to any changes, any possible improvements, I sit and wonder about its mysterious effects. Am I any different? Are things a little clearer? Would I recognise it if they were? I am still in the novelty stage, it feels shiny and new, a gimmick, and I like it. I like to tell myself that if it isn't noticeably working yet, it will tomorrow, or the day after. Maybe it is working right now, and I just don't see it.

They – and I am not sure who *they* are; just random people, probably – they say that there are five stages to loss and grief. There is denial and anger. There is bargaining and depression. And there is acceptance.

I have been ill a long while now, almost two years. I'm a veteran. I have experienced the loss of my health and grief for its passing, and I have gone through the subsequent denial and anger (isolation, too). I may be in the bargaining stage now, and for all I know depression looms, but greater in my field of vision at the moment, I think, is acceptance, or something like it. It has taken some time to get here, but it could hardly have arrived any quicker, if only because these things take time. The acceptance seems to be coinciding with the meditation, or perhaps the meditation is helping me with the acceptance. I could have started meditating two years ago – the offer was there – but I didn't feel ready for it then. The fact that I do now must have something to do with this fifth stage. And so I am not entirely clear which it is that is making me feel better, calmer, more generally at peace, less fearful, and that has left me with a certain physical confidence restored. Is this the acceptance at work, or the meditation? Does it matter?

I cannot really grasp acceptance, it is too intangible, too in the ether; but meditation is more definable, there are classes for it, apps. So I go with the meditation. And Headspace has piqued my interest. I want to do more of it, but I want now to research what else is out there, to browse the competition, the alternatives, in the hope that one appeals more than all the others, that one goes deeper, feels more thorough, is the best fit, *works*.

And then, a week later, I find it, unexpectedly one breezy Thursday evening, in SE1, just off the Tower Bridge Road, a short way down from a Tesco Metro.

Fourteen

I am standing in silence in a living room alongside a man I have just met, Will Williams. It is meant to be a contemplative, even spiritual, silence, but I spend it trying not to envy his apartment overlooking the Thames, and failing miserably. It's a converted warehouse space with exposed wooden beams and views of the river. We are facing the wall, in front of a framed picture of somebody called Guru Dev, one of the masters of the Vedic tradition. Will has his eyes closed, is singing something in what I later find out is Sanskrit, and is offering to Dev the gifts I have been encouraged to bring – three pieces of fruit and a bunch of thornless flowers, Tesco's cellophane removed. As he sings in a mellifluous, sinewy voice that would never win him a recording contract, I steal a glance at him – at Will, not Dev. His eyes are closed. He looks utterly serene.

Will Williams is more Andy Puddicombe than he is Guru Dev, the modern face of an ancient practice, with a handsome website that appeals to the curious novice like me. He wears a pale V-necked jumper and a brand of jeans I would like to own, stylish, likely expensive. He once worked in the music industry, but has left all that behind to become instead an entrepreneurial Vedic meditation master, his objective to make it everyone's meditation of choice. He runs city courses and weekend retreats at plush country manors.

After several more minutes of Sanskrit verse, he motions me to follow him in kneeling. This makes me a little uncomfortable, genuflecting before a spiritual icon I have never heard of along-side a total stranger. I plan potential escape routes, in case they prove necessary. Is the door locked, the key hidden? Then, so suddenly it takes me by surprise, Will turns towards me and whispers something directly in my ear, his breath hot and inti-mate against my skin. Though I do not know it yet, this is to be my own personal Vedic mantra, which I will say repetitively in my mind for 20 minutes twice a day, every day.

He stops. We move to the sofa, exchange a glance and smile at one another. 'That was the only really ceremonial bit,' he says reassuringly. 'Everything else is very normal, very ordinary.'

Seated close together, a cushion separating us, he requests that I close my eyes and repeat my mantra aloud, two sylla-bles that feel pleasant on the tongue. I do this for a full minute, after which he tells me to say it quieter, then as a whisper, and then eventually only in my head until I am sure I have it down and memorised.

I am to do this now for a full 20 minutes, my first proper go at Vedic. It takes an age to pass. Time slows, then trickles, to what is surely a standstill, and all the while I can sense Will a foot away on the sofa. Is he staring at me? Should I look? I cannot hear him breathe, and for a moment I wonder whether he has gone, but I think I sense the warmth of his presence on me. I feel awkward at the prospect he might be watching me, voyeuristically, and I try to put it out of my mind. I fight against the impulse to scratch, to fidget. *Focus*. I focus on my mantra, the clean crispness that encourages metronomic repetition, and gradually I begin to drift. The silence is a vacuum, an absence, but then it begins to fill me up, like a pump, until I am full with it.

Eventually, Will makes a noise that signals the end of the session, but he encourages me to keep my eyes closed for a further two minutes, thus facilitating a re-entry to consciousness with minimum disruption.

When I open my eyes, I turn to see him smiling back at me beatifically. I tell him I feel as if I have woken from a particularly deep sleep, and that I feel refreshed. The sunlight somehow seems brighter.

He beams.

'When we meditate,' he tells me, 'we achieve deep, deep rest, and the nervous system is able to spontaneously heal itself of old pain and emotion and any negative response patterns. The more we do this, the more they will wither away. We then have the freedom to make conscious choices about how to respond to life's circumstances. Occasionally, we may trick ourselves into responding according to our old patterns, but increasingly we find a better way to engage.'

He nods once at me, and I nod back at him.

'Good, then,' he says. 'See you tomorrow.'

On the way out, he gifts me two of the three pieces of fruit I had brought for the guru, another little bit of ceremony to demonstrate the warm feelings that come when we share.

Back out on the street, I peel and eat the orange. It tastes good.

Vedic meditation has been around for thousands of years. It was repressed by the British in colonial times after they became suspicious of the natives indulging in quite so rum a practice, but it was subsequently revived when the British left, and has blossomed in popularity ever since. It now boasts a global following. Vedic has a close cousin in Transcendental Meditation, both requiring the repetition of personalised mantras, and consisting of two daily sessions lasting 20 minutes. Any significant difference between the two, at least for the novice, is negligible, but TM is by far the more popular, and consequently more fashionable. The American film director David Lynch runs a foundation in America that works to make TM available to as many people as possible, and as a result it is now taught in schools, the workplace, even prisons. Celebrities have dabbled, a factor that has afforded the discipline many column inches. When I contact a TM centre in the UK, explaining that I am a journalist and wondering if it might be possible to sit in on a course, the lady I speak to groans. 'Oh no,' she says, 'not another one.' TM is popular enough. It doesn't need the likes of me to promote it further.

Vedic, then, is in its shadow. Will Williams tells me he considers it the purer form.

It is the mantra that sets both apart from other similar practices. The mantra is a set of phonemes, or vibrations, that allow the nervous system to relax, and encourage the brain to go into a state of coherence. Ordinarily, the brain is only 30–40 per cent coherent at any one time; at all other times there is too much competing white noise. This is where the mantra comes in. As one starts to repeat it, the brain begins to slow down and moves gradually into alpha state. Alpha state is something all brains unwittingly crave, because it allows the constituent parts to move towards greater coherence. Disruptive frequencies – inhibiting thoughts, anxiety – can now settle, which balances the nervous system and all the other systems within the body that have been put out of alignment by the simple toil of daily life.

'And so,' Will explains, 'on a physiological level, everything is now moving in the direction of going back to its default setting of optimal functionality.'

Will stumbled onto Vedic after he became ill in 2007. He had been managing a number of bands, putting on music events, and generally living the kind of lifestyle that is commensurate to burnout. After a trip to South America, he returned home convinced he had caught some kind of tropical disease. His liver wasn't working properly, nor his thyroid. His doctor said that he was on course for diabetes unless he quickly changed his diet, his lifestyle. He had trouble sleeping. So he stopped drinking and cleared the fridge completely of ready meals. He dabbled with reflexology, acupuncture, hypnosis; anything he could think of to help break through what was increasingly becoming a debilitating condition.

A friend suggested he try meditating. Will had grown up in East Grinstead, the cult capital of Europe, and the UK HQ for Scientologists, Mormons, Jehovah's Witnesses (it has a lot of ley lines). Growing up in such an environment had left him with an ingrained suspicion for anything even vaguely alternative, and he had already found the reflexology, the acupuncture and the hypnosis a stretch. But he was desperate, and decided to give it a go.

It worked.

'The more I meditated, the more my consciousness felt like it was expanding,' he tells me. Intrigued, he started to look into the ancient Vedic knowledge, and began reading books on the subject. 'It was blowing me away, opening up all the mysteries of the universe to me.'

As he began to feel better, the prospect of returning to his day job suddenly seemed vacuous, a waste of precious time. 'I no longer wanted to do something simply for the sake of paying the bills; that just felt irrelevant. I thought it was time to start growing personally.'

He studied Vedic for two years in the UK, but then, craving more, went to India to train with the masters. He returned, not in a robe, but convinced that what he had learned was special enough to now impart to as many people as possible, albeit in ways amenable to the Western mindset. In conversation, Will can come across as evangelical about his discoveries. His eyes shine when he talks, and he has the kind of smile you would expect of Scrabble players who have a triple word score looming. But he has dialled down the cult sensibilities, the incense whiff of overt spirituality, and there is really nothing otherworldly about him at all. The modern guru is a necessary chameleon.

'I want to teach it in a way to fully convey its benefits for people over here,' he says. 'And for me, that means: don't make it dogmatic, doctrinal. I don't want to sit here and tell people what to do and how to do it. Instead, I want to give them the tools to start accessing their most divine natures, their deepest, most expanded selves. Because once you start familiarising yourself with that at an experiential level, then maybe you'll become as connected to it as I did, and you'll want to share the richness as well. It is such a simple technique. You don't need to be told what the rules are, because you will tune into the rules yourself, and work it out for yourself. The best thing to do is to go out and experience it yourself, because once you have, there will be no more doubt in your mind as to its benefits.'

An introductory course in Vedic meditation costs several hundred pounds and takes place over four consecutive days. After my initial introduction, I return again on Friday evening, this time alongside seven other beginners. Most are in their 30s or 40s, one is a little younger, another much older. I am sitting next to a man with a shaved head, a lot of bulk, and tattoos on his forearms that his Stone Island shirt fails to conceal. He looks like he knows about anger, and how to wield it, and his faltering smile does nothing to minimise the aura of menace. But he proves, over time, to be a sweet man, and intensely vulnerable. At least once every session, seemingly unprompted, he begins to sweat profusely and to tremble, the mild tremors of a panic attack. It is at this point that he no longer looks capable of great violence, but rather like he is about to burst into copious tears.

On the other side of me is a woman, a yoga teacher. She tells us she has a hole in her heart, and that she recently had a stroke. Doctors have told her to expect another one soon. She used to love to paint, but is unable to now. Another woman, the oldest here and originally from the Caribbean, tells us that she has been living with pain for many years. 'I'm sick of being sick,' she says, and the smile she summons is purely heartbreaking. And then there is the ebullient actress, who, once she starts talking, finds she cannot stop, offering meandering explanations, then apologies for them, then falls into a self-conscious giggle and an all-enveloping laugh. She is in her mid-40s, she has multiple sclerosis, and is currently between relationships, flat-sharing with someone she doesn't like. She talks on, entertaining everyone, until Will gently clears his throat. He explains that during each meditation session, we will be expelling all sorts of toxins. This might send some of us plummeting in an emotional freeall, but if it does, do not worry. It's temporary.

Will sits at the far end of the room, with us gathered in front of him in a semi-circle. Behind him are two large windows that open onto a balcony which overlooks a small inlet of river and, beyond that, another grand warehouse building converted into apartments. Our view is of dozens of floor-to-ceiling windows offering views into dozens of separate lives. At 7.30 in the evening, it proves better than watching television, people arriving home from work as one by one the darkened windows suddenly flood with light. As Will explains that, via regular practice, we will begin to feel more energised, invigorated, confident and playful, I watch a man over his left shoulder, in his bedroom, wearing nothing but a very tight pair of bright red briefs, begin his yoga routine. Even from this distance, his abs are clearly defined. I sneak a look at the actress; she is watching him, too.

A light in the next apartment goes on. A couple, dressed in suits. She carelessly discards her handbag, he his newspaper, and the actress and I watch as they move into the curtainless bedroom and get undressed. They let their clothes fall where they stand, then reach for T-shirts and sweatpants. Back in the other room, the woman opens the large fridge and takes out two or three boxes, last night's takeaway perhaps, which she hands to him, before turning back for cutlery and a bottle of wine, a pair of wine glasses. Together they sit on the sofa, the backs of their heads to us, and eat while watching TV.

'. . . So let's do that now,' Will is saying. 'Ready? Close your eyes.'

I am grateful for the distraction, and for the next 20 minutes we meditate in an eerie collective silence, the very fact of being surrounded by other people doing exactly what I am doing lending the practice an atmosphere so physical I feel I could reach out and touch it.

We meet again just 12 hours later, early – arguably too early – on Saturday morning, and then again on Sunday. During the sessions, each of which lasts three hours, Will gives us a very thorough overview of the practice's origins and of the myriad benefits of becoming a practitioner ourselves. Each of these benefits he backs up, at length, with reference to scientific corroboration. He speaks of the infinite reservoirs of energy, vitality, creativity and wisdom that run in all of us, and how all we need to do to become our optimal selves is to learn how to access them. Meditation promotes increased activity in the prefrontal cortex of the brain, which is where we experience our high-level thinking. If we meditate regularly, then we will enter further into the realms of pure consciousness.

'If you are able to de-excite your nervous system to such a profound level that it can then tune into the underlying field of consciousness, then you are able to tune into all sorts of different layers, and go deep,' he says.

He tells us that, after years of practice, he himself has reached higher states of consciousness. I ask him what it was like.

'Wow,' is his reply, eyes like saucers.

Occasionally over the weekend, one of us will forget our personalised mantra, at which point Will, falling into ceremony again, leads us into another room to re-whisper it in our ears. I read later, online, that such privacy is to preserve the original effectiveness and purity of the technique. If the mantras are not carefully safeguarded, shrouded in their mystical secrecy, then that purity might become diluted, their effectiveness lost. That at least is the claim.

It's one way to keep TM teachers in business.

We complete the daily sessions with our 20 minutes of collective silence, each of us mentally intoning our mantras, not a sound in the room save for the percussive rumblings of stomachs, because when one rumbles, another inevitably follows, like yawns. At the end of each, Will brings us back into the here and now, his apartment with its exposed beams and river views, a benevolent smile on his face as he offers us more herbal tea.

'You will all see a lot of changes over the next few months,' he predicts. 'Keep in touch, let me know how you get on.'

The yoga teacher, the woman with the hole in her heart, has questions. She drills him on the finer points of the science of it, and there is much discussion of the toxin release. Will she, she wants to know, shout at her husband again, like she did last night?

'If you do, it's natural, it's normal,' Will assures her. 'And don't worry, it will pass.'

And this is how it finishes. I have found it fascinating and invigorating, and I have enjoyed it more than I might have expected. Will is a persuasive teacher. I do wonder how much of it I have really taken in, but this doesn't matter because what I am left with – that there is ample scientific proof that meditation is no mere fad or gimmick but something that actually works, and has worked for millions of people over thousands of years – resonates powerfully. And I like doing it, I like the idea of two sessions per day, the prolonged, almost taunting silence it requires from an individual, the concentration, a certain mettle, even. I want to do this – more than mindfulness, more than yoga nidra – again.

I glance around the room. Everybody looks hopeful and enthused. We hug one another before we leave, and then we disperse into the winding, maze-like streets of Shad Thames. Elena had brought me here earlier by car, but now I walk. The sun is out, its glare bouncing off the harsh metallic sheen of the river. I stop at a café, where I plan to eat a light salad but order instead a large arancini ball, a cluster of rice deep-fried in breadcrumbs and filled with Bolognese sauce. While I work my way through it, I reach over and pick up the newspaper that has been left on the next table. Inside, I find a four-page article on Andy Puddicombe extolling the many wonders of meditation. How strange, I think. Coincidence or kismet? I resume my walk along the river, then up and over Tower Bridge, and onto a bus that takes me towards an East London market I used to visit regularly but now haven't seen in three years. I feel unusually calm and, if not quite serene – never that, not me – then happy and hopeful that something has been invigorated within me. Just being here, out, alone, so far from home – all this is novelty. The market has undergone faceless regeneration in my absence, but the terrific bookstall is still here. I buy a book, then browse the other stalls on the way to meet Elena and the girls, who are waiting patiently for me in the car by the Tube station. Even simply doing this – *me* walking to *them* instead of them coming to fetch me – is new, a minor miracle. I find it difficult not to grin foolishly, a baby taking its first uncertain steps. Elena sees me through the windscreen, her smile so full of encouragement a lump comes to my throat.

It is a long day, and it should deplete me considerably, leaving me wiped out for at least the next week. But somehow it doesn't. Somehow, I very nearly feel fine. Odd.

Is it working, then?

The answer to that is: yes, it is – to a point. But I have become so accustomed to my new, gradually changing reality that I still frequently fail to recognise it. Progress comes in fits and starts, full of one-step-forward-two-steps-back lurches that test my patience, mock my optimism and unravel my resolve. Bluntly put, I'm still knackered most of the time, quite spectacularly knackered, and still fearful that whatever I do to push my parameters will knacker me more.

Though this condition feels so palpably physical, targeting my by now weak muscles, I am increasingly aware of the mental grip it has on me. I want to get back out there again, I really do, but everywhere I look I see reminders of places where I have tried and failed, familiar roads which I can no longer manage, the impossibility of my getting from A to B without paying for it severely afterwards. There are too many memories here. I've no option, though, but to try. Because walking still seems to take so much out of me – the post-Vedic high on which I'd strolled through the market soon faded – and because the silent fear of it doing so ratchets up my cortisol to unhelpful levels, those times I do venture outside, I cycle. Cycling, I find, is easier, and requires less effort. I cycle the girls to and from school each day, and cycle to my local café for an afternoon break, where I sit still half-bewildered that I have managed the journey at all, and that I am actually outside among people. The amount of mental planning this all requires is considerable, and has forced me to become a kind of mathematician, forever working out the likely distance of every outdoor undertaking, and how I can undertake it with the minimum effort possible. On jobs into town, I cycle to the train station, the train takes me into the centre, and then, necessarily avoiding the mocking labyrinth of the Tube, I head instead towards the nearest bus stop and take the first bus that comes along. This will take me to other bus stops, at least one of which I will be able to change at and await another that will take me closer to my destination. All of this, it goes without saying, will have been pre-planned online the night before. If the distance from the bus stop to my eventual destination is sufficiently close, I will brave the final walk there; if not, I will have scouted out the nearest Boris bike docking station, and undertake the final leg on two wheels.

Either way, I arrive at my destination a little wired and greatly relieved. This is improvement, emphatically so, and I need to remind myself of it repeatedly. I ignore the still-present sensation of fatigue because, look, here I am, out in the world again and interacting with others, and I sit down to interview the person I have come to meet looking to all intents and purposes just as they seem to me: capable, ordinary, normal.

We start heading further afield at the weekends, too, into other parts of town – visiting shops, browsing markets, different parks – the change of scenery so much better than my habitual rest. I never accompany my family all the way, usually bailing out, puffing, at the nearest café in order to allow them to wander at will, because they are people who don't count their footsteps, nor do they fear what those footsteps will bring.

Each Sunday outing ends the same way. The moment we get home, I make my way upstairs and attempt to meditate for up to 20 minutes, in the hope of lowering the cortisol currently firing around my system, and keen to calm the sense of foreboding at the now rapidly unfurling exhaustion climbing up my legs like vines and weighing with heavy familiarity across my shoulders and back.

It is impossible not to be acutely aware of just how palpably bad I feel at these times, but I know that this is the very time I am supposed to say my STOP!s, loudly and repeatedly in my head, in order to break the destructive thought patterns circling on a loop, and instead be returned to the moment, mindfully and meditatively, as instructed.

But this is where, for me, it becomes confusing. To be in the moment is to realise how I am feeling right now, which is dreadful, which leads inevitably to the concrete conviction that I will pay dearly for my exertions well into the following week. I mustn't think like this, and so I STOP! once more, barring those intrusive thoughts and re-focusing on the here and now, but the here and now is clouded with heady fatigue, so – *STOP!*

And so, yet again, I STOP!, with a Tourette's-like tenacity, a hamster in a wheel going nowhere fast, hoping against what feels like pointless hope that this is all merely temporary, that I will get through this eventually, and that, if nothing else, it is character building. Long term, I say to myself with a mostly straight face, this will probably do me the world of good, make me a better person. Right?

Fifteen

I plough on. The Vedic high may have settled, as all highs must, but the shift it effects within me lingers on. It does. It is a subtle shift, but I gradually accept that life is nevertheless inching back towards that elusive state of normal, and in its slipstream I resume ordinary citizenship. I bin the taxi-firm cards that come through the letterbox most mornings, assured I no longer have use for them, and delete their numbers from my phone. I invest in an Oyster card. I am out of the house more, freer. I am a veteran of this thing, almost two years now, but I am in recovery. If someone suggests we meet up, I am more likely to go.

'You're looking well' is something I occasionally hear from the few friends I have left. They had expected, not unreasonably, to see evidence of the condition that had taken me out of the game, only to find me looking much the same. They are confused, but then they are not the only ones. The truth is I haven't really handled the friend situation particularly well. I didn't know how to. Just because I have always failed in sustaining those alpha male friendships in which conversation revolves around girls and football and cars doesn't make me automatically comfortable in discussing my failing health with beta equivalents. I never know quite how to broach the subject, aware that it's a mood killer, and so I don't. And on those few occasions I try, I fail to relay the gravity of the situation. After telling one friend about it a month on from the initial diagnosis, she called the following week asking if I fancied going out for drinks. I tried to explain that my problem was more long term, that I wouldn't be going out for drinks for some considerable time. I barely heard from her again. And to the old friend upon whom I unburdened myself one night – feeling it appropriate to respond in kind after he had told me of his own troubles (largely marital) – he responded with what I thought was understanding, but then asked whether I was still cycling all over town and travelling regularly. Elsewhere, I resolved simply never to broach the topic at all with friends, and if they did, to summarise with an editor's eye for the succinct, and move on.

We live in a world where we mostly get well soon or else we very dramatically don't. If you occupy the uncertain middle ground, then it all gets invariably confusing. My oldest, and closest, friend empathised better than most, and accepted unquestioningly that things were suddenly very different for me now. She would make the effort to come and see me, and if we did meet in town, insisted on paying for the taxi home. She could not, of course, have realised that something far more dramatic was about to befall her, but when it did I was quick to respond in kind.

She was standing in her front garden one July morning pruning plants when she experienced what she later said felt like a heavy shovel smacking the back of her head. She collapsed to the ground, her three-month-old puppy confusing it all for a game. Her neighbour called an ambulance. My friend's husband called me a day later, exhausted and emotionally spent, the unavoidable consequence of having to go through their address book and contact all her close friends to explain that she had had a brain haemorrhage, had almost died and may never fully recover, that the rehabilitation process would be slow and draining, and that she would not be fit for visitors for several weeks, possibly months.

Here was a proper death-dodging drama that put my problem in its long shadow. It was months before I saw her again, her husband necessarily over-protective and under doctor's orders to keep her away from too much noise, too much light, too much activity, and children under the age of 10. She had neurological damage, and possible memory problems; she would require monitoring for the next several years. She was told that the life she had been living, an otherwise eminently ordinary urban adult life, was now too much for her. She needed emphatic change.

To my surprise, she did as she was told. A brain haemorrhage can have a chastening effect. She left London for the coast, her job for art therapy and, much later, Open University courses, and the daily commute for long walks on an empty beach with the dog, whose constant presence was likely key to her ongoing recovery. She was still the same person, and looked the same, but she had fundamentally changed. She stopped drinking, severed certain ties, and sought only tranquillity. Friends became a drain on her remaining resources, family members too. They didn't much like this new incarnation, and even after patient explanation could never fully comprehend that the change was permanent, the ramifications of this considerable.

'But it's been two years,' friends would say. She began screening her calls.

Her illness has brought us closer, even as geography has kept us apart. No more do we meet up every couple of weeks in pursuit of morning-after hangovers, and when we do get together, we observe strict codes of conduct our younger selves would never have seen coming. Her brain has been damaged, and so she requires handling with care: no noise, no alcohol, zero caffeine, a pass on dessert, an early night.

There is gallows humour to be found here, buckets of it. We find it because we have to.

*

The woman on my PC screen is telling me something that makes me sit up straight.

'I'm going to communicate with your super-conscious mind now,' she says.

She is doing this in an attempt to make me better, to cure me, via a process called Psych-K. No one has ever attempted to communicate with my super-conscious mind before. I am intrigued. But there is something called a permission protocol to go through first.

'We never assume it's okay to make changes, because there might be consequences,' she explains. 'We always have to check with the higher self that it is safe and appropriate, that it means no harm, that it's in your best interest.'

She does this now by asking my super-conscious mind for permission to proceed. The objective here is to find out why the burnout I suffered, which left behind such long-standing consequences, occurred. The woman, whom I shall call Lucinda, says she might be able to fix me.

We are conversing via Skype. If we were meeting in person, she says, she would be doing muscle testing on me, or kinesiology, which is the study of the mechanics of body testing, a procedure that aims to find imbalances within the body by getting to the root of the problem, be it physical, chemical, emotional or, according to one website I encounter, 'energetical'. There are several different strands of kinesiology, but at the heart of each lies the theory of muscle testing. Muscle testing involves testing a particular body part, usually the arm, for strength or weakness. The stronger it is, the more conviction in the belief; the weaker, the less. We have over 640 muscles in our body, all connected to different organs via neural pathways. By applying pressure to a muscle to gauge its response, a practitioner is able to read bio-feedback within that organ's meridian, and so uncover the underlying causes of health problems and

their symptoms. Treatment includes nutritional recommendations, acupuncture, lymphatic massage and emotional support.

Because we cannot do normal muscle testing over the internet,
Lucinda tells me she is able to substitute it with something just
as effective: a pendulum. The pendulum will rotate clockwise if
my super-consciousness conveys strength and conviction, anti-
clockwise if not.

Now Lucinda asks the higher self: 'Is it safe and appropriate
for Nick to learn the messages and start to release his fatigue?'
The pendulum is held up before her at eye level. It swings confi-
dently clockwise.

'Lovely,' she says. Permission protocol has been granted, just
like that.

'Is Nick consciously aware of what the message is?' she asks.
The pendulum now swings anti-clockwise. 'No,' she says.

Earlier in our conversation, she had asked me about my life,
my upbringing, my experiences as a child, events around the
time I first fell ill. Now she asks of the pendulum: 'Is the message
connected to Nick's experiences as a child?' It swings clockwise. 'Yes. So there is a connection here. Is there,' she asks, 'any
significance to the timing?' The pendulum swings anti-clockwise. 'No, it could have happened at any time.'

Another question. 'Are there beliefs associated with Nick's
fatigue at this point in his life?'

Clockwise.

'Yes. There are subconscious beliefs that have brought this on.'

She looks up from the pendulum, and at me. 'Let me know
if any of this gets confusing,' she says. 'Or if you simply think,
What on earth is she talking about?' I nod. 'Is Nick aware of what
those beliefs are?'

Anti-clockwise.

'Okay, so the protocol now is to find out where to go next.
I am communicating with your entire system here,' she points

out. 'I'm not deciding myself what it is because I don't know; I can't possibly know what's best for you. But I am communicating with your system, and it tells me that every part of your system is ready, willing and able to balance, and to begin to completely recover from fatigue.'

I want to ask her: *Yes, but how?*, when our Skype connection is lost. She calls back moments later, and is now holding a large book in her hand, A4-size. This book, she explains, contains 1,500 belief statements in it.

'I am communicating with your higher self, and it is going to guide us to the first belief you need to change, and that can help you to start recovering.'

I want to ask her *How?* again, but remain silent.

'We have no idea what is coming,' she says, adding, 'This is fun. It may not make conscious sense, but this is what is going on at a deep level. You can't be aware of it consciously, and you would probably only ever be able to do so if you went into therapy, but right now we are talking to your *core*.'

She starts leafing through the pages quickly for my appropriate belief statement.

'It's between pages 20 and 30, between 20 and 25, 26 and 30.' Still she leafs. 'Page 27, 28, page 29, page 30. Your belief is on page 30.' I register here a rush of emotion. We are closing in on it, whatever *it* may be. 'The category is Fun, Play and Adventure. I wonder,' she says, 'if when you were younger, you allowed yourself to be a child.'

I think the question is rhetorical, so I say nothing, but after a moment's silence, Lucinda looking intently at me on my screen, I answer. Yes, I say, I think I did.

'Let's see what comes up, then. Your belief statement is between numbers one and 10, it's between 11 and 20, between 16 and 20. The priority belief statement is number 16, number 17, number 18, number 19, number 20.' Her finger, travelling down the page, stops abruptly. 'It is statement number 20: I Am Fun to Be With.'

She looks up at me. I nod: okay.

'How does that sound? Does it make any sense? Do you feel you are fun to be around?

I tell her yes.

'Okay then, let's test that belief. Let's see if you believe it unconsciously.'

When you do muscle testing, Lucinda explains, you assume a posture: feet parallel on the floor, eyes looking down but not closed, not straining them. I assume the posture.

'Now say it out loud: *I am fun to be with*. Say it like you really mean it.'

I do. The pendulum swings anti-clockwise.

I tell Lucinda that the pendulum is wrong. I *am* fun to be with. I am!

'What this means,' she says, possibly trying to soothe, 'is that you probably do think you are fun to be with but that your current belief is that you are not.'

'Due to the extenuating circumstances?' I say.

'Well, possibly, yes. There is some kind of push/pull here. You have to try a little harder to have fun, to be fun, and to align your subconscious beliefs with your conscious goal.'

This is all linked, she stresses, to the fatigue. If I manage to rewire my belief, she says, 'then things could open up for you, this could be the start of the process of you getting better.'

She tells me to cross my ankles, and does a little kinesiology, via the pendulum, as to which ankle I should cross over which. The pendulum suggests left over right. She tells me to entwine my hands, cross them at the wrist, then turn them inside out and bring them up underneath my chin. This crossing over of limbs, she says, is a way of activating both hemispheres of the brain. When you do this, the subconscious mind cannot hold the resistance of the change for longer than two to five minutes, and allows the system to relax.

I am now to repeat my belief – *I am fun to be with* – silently, over and over.

'The subconscious mind likes familiarity, so because it currently believes you are not fun to be with, then it stops you from really fulfilling the ability to be so. This will undo it.'

She explains that somewhere inside of two to five minutes, there will be a change. The way I say the words might change, or there might be a physical change, a yawn perhaps, or else a sense of relaxation throughout the body. There could even be an emotional change. I might start laughing, crying.

'It's different for every person. You might not even be aware of the changes as they occur.'

I close my eyes and repeat my belief. *I am fun to be with, I am fun to be with, I am fun to be with*. She tells me to continue to say it until I have experienced a mental, physical or emotional change, some indication that the resistance to the belief has evaporated, gone.

'And when you do feel ready, open your eyes. Take as long as it takes.'

After a while, perhaps closer to two minutes and certainly not as many as five, I open my eyes. Lucinda swings the pendulum to test whether it has worked, the belief reversed. It swings anti-clockwise.

'It's not complete. The change hasn't happened fully yet. We are experiencing some resistance. But don't worry, it's all completely normal. Let's repeat it again.'

She encourages me to think back to a time in my life when I was both having fun and being fun. I do this now, running a succession of memories in my head. The process is pleasant, like the positive visualisation exercises I have been doing. When I open my eyes, Lucinda seems excited. She is grinning.

'When I looked at you while you were doing it,' she says, 'you had a very serene smile on your face, and I could see your whole body relaxing, your shoulders dropping. So let's see if it has worked.'

She holds up the pendulum. It swings clockwise.

'A lovely big clockwise rotation this time! Which means that you now fully believe the statement 100 per cent. You have shifted the resistance. Well done.'

Weeks earlier, I had emailed a man called Rob Williams, the creator of Psych-K, an international operation of which Lucinda is one of the European representatives. I explained my situation. I wrote that I had come across him during my research, and felt that Psych-K sounded interesting, and perhaps worth investigating further, with a view to writing about it.

He wrote a sympathetic letter back, suggesting that he understood my disappointment in trying to deal with such a diagnosis from a mainstream medical point of view. He didn't believe they had much to offer me, given their belief in the 'reductionist medical model'. From their perspective, he wrote, all disease has a physical basis only, which leaves the mind out of the equation. Psych-K recognises the mind and the spirit of an individual as integral components of any disease process. He attached an interview he had recently given that explained his philosophy about disease and healing, and said he would like to know more about my book before agreeing to be a part of it. Psych-K, he said, is a bit like swimming: you can't really know it without a direct experience. He concluded his letter: 'As Einstein once said, "Knowledge is experience, everything else is just information."'

I looked him up. Williams was a rugged-looking American in his early 60s, a psychotherapist whose objective had been to combine the worlds of business and counselling. He had wanted to find more effective treatments to help clients make positive changes in their lives, and over the years he had studied neurolinguistic programming, hypnosis, a practice called Touch for Health, reiki and kinesiology.

Psych-K was something he developed out of his extensive studies of these alternative practices. In the interview he referenced, he spoke of how the subconscious directs the body's motor functions and controls muscle movements. What Psych-K does is to use the musculature in order to communicate with the subconscious. It's like a lie-detector test. A lie-detector test measures skin conductivity. When somebody is telling a lie, they become tense, their blood pressure rises, which makes them sweat and increases skin conductivity. Measuring differences in muscle tension can lead to similar results.

Williams wasn't a self-help guru or a quack (Lucinda would later tell me that he never believed he created Psych-K: 'He just tuned into it, he meditated, and the information came to him'). If you like the sound of all this, Williams seemed to be saying, fine; if not, 'bye. There was no Psych-K advertising campaign, no hard sell.

'If we decide that including Psych-K in your book is a good idea, then a direct experience is in order, so you can speak from your own experience, not mine,' he wrote in his email to me.

Which is how I come to be speaking to Lucinda today, one weekday mid-morning, while her young son is at nursery. She is sweet and cheery and self-deprecating.

She tells me a little more about the practice and its ethos, which is simply to change negative, self-limiting beliefs. 'It's like peeling the layers of an onion,' she says. 'I know it's a stereotypical analogy, but it works. We start off by peeling the top layers of belief, which allows the deep stuff that has been pushed down to come up. Eventually you get to the core to find nothing else to work with.' She smiles. 'It's a journey.'

She tells me that she is a veteran of my condition herself, all better now, and how so many people these days are perhaps guilty of over-managing their lives too much. We talk about self-protection, and how self-protection is very often the problem. Whichever problem we have, be it mental, physical or spiritual, the philosophy behind it is that the problem is a separation from our higher self, our own divinity, our higher consciousness.

If I'm honest, I have trouble grasping all that she says, but she says it with such clear-eyed conviction. I do not consider her cuckoo.

'The subconscious is a million times more powerful than the conscious. So this is where we have to make the changes, in our subconscious, not our conscious minds. In this way we can be absolutely aligned with our higher purpose – if, that is, you want to talk about it in those terms. In other words, the things we want most in our lives are the things we have to believe in subconsciously as well as consciously.'

Making changes in our conscious mind is all very well, she goes on, but this can quite often be draining and energy-consuming in itself. Plus, our subconscious can quite easily overtake these efforts and render them redundant anyway. 'Ninety-five per cent of our lives is driven by subconscious programming,' she says.

The belief statements we are working on are not unlike positive affirmations, but, accessed via Psych-K, they go deeper.

'We use your body to communicate with them to get a read-out of what's really going on.'

How? I ask her. She explains more about muscle testing.

'We can use any muscle in your body, but generally we use the arm. We press down on the arm. So you would say, for example, My name is Nick. We press down on your arm, and it will lock, just stop. But if we said your name was Celia, there would be confusion in your subconscious mind, and the arm would go weak.' She pauses. 'Are you following me?'

I nod, yes.

'It's electrical impulses in the brain, essentially. They are firing off into the body whenever the brain and body communicate. The electrical impulses are being driven by the subconscious mind. When you say something that is true, those impulses in the brain stay strong. But when you lie, the subconscious mind gets confused. The impulses fire off in the brain, there is massive confusion, and by the time we get to the muscles in the body, the strength in those muscles has weakened. That's why the arm cannot hold, and lock, in place.'

(Later, I try this out for myself, keen to try the muscle rather than the pendulum. I find that my arm is able to lock on both Nick and Celia. Either I am doing it wrong, or else I have pathological tendencies.)

I ask the obvious question: during the testing via Skype, isn't she directly responsible for which way the pendulum swings?

Her smile does not waver. 'Does it look like I'm swinging it in one direction or the other?'

I have to admit that, no, it doesn't.

'What we are trying to do here is to bring you out of your thoughts and beliefs about over-protection. You were ill, but you're not any more. We need to look at what else is going on inside you, at an emotional level.'

I should use this as an opportunity for self-development, she says. Health conditions often force us to re-evaluate our lives. In other words, there are lessons to be learned.

It is at this point that she says she is going to communicate with my super-conscious mind. I sit forward and give her my full attention.

We start the process again, Lucinda flicking through the pages, looking for another belief to test out. She goes now from page 20 to 30, and announces that it is between 30 and 41, 41 and

50, 51 and 59. I find myself wondering what is driving her on through the pages. Is she really somehow communicating with my higher self via an internet connection, and is my higher self really somehow communicating back the page at which she should stop? If so, how? And who has written these particular beliefs? And why? And are they really quite so easy to unlock?

'It's between 55 and 59,' she is saying, then: 'Page 56. Success and Achievement.' Again I register a thrill of anticipation. I cannot wait to hear what she is about to reveal. 'The statement is: *Success and achievement are natural outcomes for me.*' She glances up at me. 'What do you think of that statement? Does it make sense?'

I laugh, and briefly tell her of all the magazines I worked on that folded, the newspapers whose arts sections continually diminish, and say that I cannot remember the last time I had a pay rise. I rarely have more than £10 credit on my Oyster card. Success and achievement, then, are hardly natural outcomes.

'So effort is needed?' she presses.

'Absolutely.'

And so we decide to amend it. Or rather, she does. She asks which belief I would like to work on instead, and then, because I really don't know what to say, she helps out. 'How about: *I have absolute and complete confidence in my abilities?*' I say that I like this one better, and so I assume the pose and repeat the belief for somewhere between two and five minutes. I open my eyes, and she swings the pendulum. Anti-clockwise. 'Repeat the process,' she instructs. I do, and now it swings clockwise.

We do not have much time left in our session, and she soon has to leave to pick up her son from the nursery. We try one final belief: that I can fully heal myself, that I have all the tools to recover my former health.

The process begins again, the closing of the eyes, the belief repeated in my mind, and then the pendulum, which at first swings (by now predictably) anti-clockwise, requiring me to repeat the process, after which it swings the other way, an indication of success.

Lucinda begins on her conclusion. 'What we have done here is identified some beliefs. You have changed them. This you must visualise every day. Really visualise them. When we want change in our lives, we can have goals, but we need to take positive action, and steps, in order to achieve that, yes?'

She says that she will make some notes for me, things for me to do, a kind of homework, and will email them, and that maybe we can do more sessions, paid sessions, this first one having been free, a generous taster.

I am a little unclear about what precisely has occurred this morning. Did I really, subconsciously, not consider myself fun, only to then fairly effortlessly reverse this thought in a few minutes? Can she really improve my health, mental and physical, in this way?

But I am intrigued, and I like her. She seems sincere, and I am interested in giving this a go because, frankly, why not?

So I wait for her email, but it never arrives. I do not hear from Lucinda again.

Sixteen

Months previously, the physiotherapist I had visited, the woman with the healing hands who had once planned on becoming a doctor, had told me how it was essential I believe I can get better. The right mindset is everything. She neglected to tell me how I might develop this belief in a world full of contradiction, and so for a long time I didn't, I couldn't. But I believe it now. You try everything, then you pick and choose, and focus on the form of therapy that you feel works best. You tune out all the competing voices, you avoid Google, and instead allow the confidence you have mustered within yourself to lead you through. It takes time to adapt to this new world, and I have a sense I will be adapting for a long while yet, but it *is* attainable. The trick is to hold on to it.

Working through this succession of therapies suits me. I like the conveyor-belt motion of it all, the next, and the next, and the next after that, in the hope that one of them might just prove to be, in inverted commas, 'it'. Therapists might call these my building blocks. With each one I register another slight improvement, more tools in my armament, and I'm happy. Every time I stumble upon one that doesn't work for me, like the lugubrious fatigue specialist who, when I spoke to him, sounded so catastrophically bored by the very subject in which he specialises that it seemed impossible he could ever really help, I simply shrug, cross it off the list and move on to the next one. My determination is steely. It is possible, of course, that I have always possessed steely determination, but am only recognising it now.

What's the opposite of catastrophising? Perhaps that's what I'm doing. I resolve to continue.

One train and two buses take me, one bright, cold Saturday morning, to East London, where, towards the end of an illuminating day, I find myself indulging in a freeform dance to the accompaniment of something called F**k It music, which is part of the whole so-called F**k It movement. The music is loud and pulsing and hypnotically repetitive. Afterwards, I will wonder if that was really me in there, shaking my melons and wilfully losing control of my limbs, but context is everything. At the time, it all seemed entirely sensible.

I am not the only one free-forming. There are about 40 of us here for a seminar entitled Let Go. It is taking place in an ugly office block one floor up from the Centre for Islamic Guidance, in a large room in which a fat tabby cat roams proprietorially. Here, we are each in the deeply private process of disrobing our inhibitions and doing something general consensus tells us we don't do anywhere enough of these days: really tuning into ourselves, to the core we all too often ignore. When we do, what do we feel? And when we do follow these core instincts – and our core instincts speak to us for a reason – what happens then?

The answer we are encouraged to come to is that we feel freer, better, liberated. Liberation is all too short-lived a sensation, says John C. Parkin, the man behind F**k It, but it doesn't have to be.

'When I first came up with the idea,' he tells me, 'it felt like magic, really. Just say fuck it to all sorts of situations, and see what happens. The fact that it works as a therapeutic tool is, to me, mind-blowing.'

The idea initially came to Parkin a decade ago, almost as a whim. But the whim had substance, and went on to become a phenomenon. Parkin has now written three books on his pet subject – *F**k It: The Ultimate Spiritual Way*, *F**k It Therapy*, and *The Way of F**k It* – which between them have sold 500,000 copies worldwide, and been translated into 22 languages. The week-long F**k It courses he runs with his wife Gaia in her native Italy are very popular, with people coming from all over the world to attend. Many return home, Parkin suggests to me, completely transformed.

Before the free-form dancing, I fall into conversation with one of my fellow attendees, a young woman called Holly, who works in marketing. She is here, she tells me, on the recommendation of a colleague. The colleague was an angry woman, 'like, all the time, a total nightmare to work with. But then she went on one of these courses, and came back completely chilled. Amazing, no?'

Holly seems utterly laid-back to me, and she emits an enviable calm, but the woman is a stranger, so what do I know? At one point during the day, we are encouraged to write down things that frustrate us in life. Holly (which is not her real name, incidentally, and she doesn't work in marketing) writes down: *Still being single. My boss. My parents.*

The Let Go seminar is essentially a pick 'n' mix self-help selection of what is covered in much more depth during the week-long retreats. It is aimed at the mildly curious, a litmus test for those wanting to pursue more thorough, and lasting, ways to evoke personal change and growth. Over the course of six hours, with an hour's break for lunch, it touches on the principles of yoga, qigong and meditation. Parkin quotes Jung, Freud and R.D. Laing, and expounds upon concepts such as high-functioning and multi-levelled consciousness. Some people take notes; all listen, rapt. He demonstrates kinesiology, and he introduces it by saying it is how 'we can all tap into our subconscious to find out what we really believe, how we restrict ourselves, and how we can learn to let go. This truth makes us stronger, and this has a huge impact on our well-being.'

I am eager to see muscle testing up close, in real life as it were, no pendulum in sight. But I am to be disappointed by it, for among the 40 of us at least, the results prove inconclusive. None of us seem quite able to get the hang of it. We are instructed to extend an arm and hold it firmly, then repeat – in our heads only – first a belief, then a lie. As Lucinda had already told me, the arm is supposed to remain firm with the belief, less so with the lie. What is interesting here is that we all want it to work, a collective willingness to witness a miracle and experience the ramifications such new knowledge might mean to us. Concerned for our health, our states of mind, each of us wants to swallow Parkin's wisdom whole and immediately reap the benefits. And so, perhaps unavoidably, we tend to make our arms stronger during the truth, if only to confirm the theory. The next time, we try to do it properly. But then, gradually, two by two – for we have teamed up in pairs – we begin to confess to doubts. Is it really working? Are our muscles really more tense when we tell the truth than when we lie? Holly, my partner, isn't fully convinced, and neither am I.

Parkin starts to explain it a little more, but time is short, he has much more ground to cover, and so we move on.

The 40 of us in attendance – Parkin calls us fuckateers – have brought so much baggage with us, it's a wonder there is any space to sit down. But we do, on the floor, crossing legs like in a school assembly, and sitting up straight. Collectively, we are dealing with the usual calamity of ordinary life: relationship issues, work crises, ill health. One man speaks of, and freely displays, anger issues that, he says, particularly come to the fore when he is behind the wheel of a car. 'And I get violent.'

Perhaps in a show of fraternity, a man across the other side of the room explains that cucumbers can make him very, very cross. Everybody laughs. A woman in her late 30s worries that her critical parents are affecting her personal relationships. She has been seeing a divorced man for three years, and is terrified that by introducing him to her parents the relationship will sour. I am surprised by how many are happy to talk to the room, out loud, in so intimate a way. One young woman, from Yorkshire, with punk hair and an Iggy Pop T-shirt, tells us about difficulties at work.

At first she hesitates, but then she says: 'Oh, I'll never see you lot again, so what difference does it make?' She says that she works in fashion, an environment where she has to look as good as possible, 'not in clothes like these, of course, and with more make-up.' But she frequently feels she falls short: 'that I'm not good enough, that I'm not pretty enough; I'm too fat'.

Some here have previous experience with alternative therapies and self-help courses, while others have been tempted through the door simply by the use of the rude word. 'F**k It sounded like a right laugh,' a young man I'll call Sav tells me. We range in age from early 20s to late 50s, *Guardian* readers mostly. There are several ruminative beards, and a lot of pseudo-tribal tattoos, but fewer sandals than one might expect. The sense of anything remotely New Age is largely conspicuous by its absence, a factor that permits many of us to unclench.

The F**k It dancing has obvious clubby comparisons, an organic equivalent to being chemically enhanced in a field somewhere outside the M25, and thus uninhibited in a way one could never be in the real world. Parkin insists it is emboldening stuff, that it peels away at the inner onions Lucinda had told me all about. He says that on his retreats, people have been known to really let go at this point, to cry, to *woof* even, and to shout out with the carefree abandon one normally associates with foreigners. Here in London, however, where most of us are diligently British, we employ a greater sense of reserve and decorum. No woofing, then, just a lot of wobbling of legs, some rocking back and forth, a few yoga poses. I keep my eyes tight shut, except when I don't, when I peek because I cannot help myself. Some look relaxed as they spin around and jump up and down on the spot, others look full of determined concentration. Few have broken out of their restricted floorspace, as if a fine might be imposed on any who dare move too freely. This isn't Italy, after all. The Yorkshire punk is making out with her boyfriend, the laying on of tantric hands. Parkin himself is performing a succession of stiff-armed robotic moves, the Tin Man dancing to Kraftwerk. I close my eyes again, face the wall and shake myself senseless.

Like taking your clothes off in public and announcing your nakedness, it is all surprisingly liberating. But then I clatter heavily into Holly, which again convinces me that one should never let oneself get too carried away in public, just in case. Health and safety.

John C. Parkin used to work in the advertising game, which probably explains his chunky zebra-striped glasses. He spent the 1990s working on campaigns for First Direct and Egg, and on mischievous ads for Pot Noodle.

'I always liked the idea of mucking around with people's heads,' he explains when we meet three days before his Let Go seminar. We are in his publisher's office in Notting Hill, a boardroom whose corner water feature strives to create an atmosphere of serenity but which instead merely sounds like a small child peeing continuously. Parkin is in his late forties, and bearded, his uncombed hair all too clearly unused to being told what to do. He boasts a belly he tells me his brother-in-law calls 'fat', and, despite living in Italy, where adherence to fashion is law, is endearingly scruffy. He looks like he's about to go rambling.

He has dabbled in yoga, Tai Chi and hypnotherapy, Christianity and, as he puts it, 'all sorts of philosophies'. He spent time in Glastonbury training to become a shamanic healer, and by 2001, he and his wife (also an alternative therapist) were parents to twin boys, and had relocated to Italy, where they started running idiosyncratic retreats in Umbria. 'HOLISTIC HOLIDAYS, ITALIAN NOSH', read their first online campaign, accompanied by a picture of a woman in yoga pose, burping loudly. The burping offended many. 'Oh, we got loads of letters saying how disgusting it was, ha ha!' he roars.

But it also attracted people turned off by other, more regimented retreats, the kind that demanded pre-dawn sessions and vows of silence and that required attendees to subsist purely on vegetables.

'I couldn't see what the problem was, starting at 10 o'clock in the morning after a hearty Italian breakfast,' he shrugs. 'And I don't see why I can't both do yoga and drink wine in the evening. Ice cream, too. I like ice cream. You know, I can do yoga, and I can also swear and get drunk at night. Does that make me any less spiritual? That was our philosophy, and people really connected to it. We weren't the only ones, in other words.'

It was at one of these early retreats that Parkin, attempting to help a Parisian businesswoman de-stress, suggested she might simply say 'fuck it' to her problems, and see what happened. This seems, on the surface, a terribly irresponsible thing to do. How much, after all, did he know of her circumstances? And how easy is it, really, to say fuck it to the job, the dog, the husband? Nevertheless, she later wrote to say how incredibly effective the advice had been. Parkin, always one to spot a potential fad, immediately realised he was onto something, and wrote his first

F**K It book, *F**K It: The Ultimate Spiritual Way*, in a frenzy. By 2008, it was an international bestseller.

The concept, he readily admits, isn't an original one. He borrowed liberally from Taoism and Buddhism, 'and all the colours of New Age spirituality'. But what he did do, and rather niftily, was to retune it to pique the interest of those people who wouldn't normally go within a mile of such books, but at the same time tap into the prevailing Zeitgeist of self-awareness, self-discovery and self-improvement. Everybody has a yoga mat these days.

Any lingering resistance people feel, he suggests, is due to its restrictive Eastern origins. But then a former adman does know how to speak to an audience, and so simply by employing that sonorous expletive, he successfully broke down any remaining barriers, and tempted the curious in their droves. Many who attend his retreats are complete newcomers.

If his books are ultimately rather silly and over-irreverent, far more concerned with making jokes than with imparting genuine enlightenment – he writes about women with 'ample breasts', of 'goat shagging', and claims that 99 per cent of all Americans are obese because they 'bin eatin' donuts again' – then in person Parkin is a much more considered, thoughtful proposition. He does not play the clown. And he presides over the Saturday seminar with an understated ease that doesn't seem to employ skill, but clearly does. He holds our attention throughout, and though he is sifting through some very edited highlights in a manner that can only ever really give us the merest hint of its true depths, it still amounts to ample food for thought. Nothing he says sounds puerile or open to ridicule. He is simply encouraging us to ask questions of ourselves, an obvious suggestion that many of us appear to overlook in the race to our daily finish lines and self-imposed deadlines. And though he himself has utilised the F**k It life to great effect – bestseller status has made him wealthy – there is nothing aggressively motivational about him as there is with so many of his peers. To me, he seems less Tony Robbins than he does Bagpuss. Listen quietly, and it is genuine wisdom he imparts.

'Are you a modern guru?' I had asked him three days previously.

'No, no, I am not,' he responded. 'I've simply been lucky enough to think about how things work and to look into the spiritual and emotional life. If anyone takes time out of their work and learns how to relax, to think about what they really want, then anyone, *everybody*, could come up with this. All I've really done is taken years out of my life to ponder it all, and I still do, six hours a day. If anything, I'm a specialist, that's all.'

I had also asked him whether he felt responsible for those who came to see him seeking answers, those he summarily sends off newly confident, and to hell with the consequences.

'No. I don't feel any responsibility at all. I just feel a joy in being able to spread these ideas, and to talk about them. I do not know more than you know. You know a lot of stuff, and you, *we*, have most of the answers within us. It's just we're not really looking. It is all there, though. It's there, but we are not listening. What we try to teach here is to give you your own sense of responsibility. What I'm trying to say is this: listen to your mind, your body. Stop holding yourself back. Put aside what society thinks about you, what *you* think about you. Instead, go inside and listen to yourself. What is it that you want? What are you thinking? What are you feeling? Your fears? Listen to the answers, and give those answers value. For many of us, we will be doing this for the first time in our lives. The more we listen, the more we relax, the more things work, the better we feel, the happier we are.'

Towards the end of the seminar, Parkin tells us to fill in the blanks in the following sentence: 'In order to feel full of . . . I need to let go of . . .' The list can be as long as we want, he says. Write as much as you like. For the next five minutes the only sound in the room is that of pen on paper, everybody scribbling furiously.

After the dance, which serves as the climax of the day, we lie down for a final meditation session. Parkin encourages us to ponder on what we have learned today, and how we might use it for quieter, less driven, more contented lives. Then it is time to go. One middle-aged woman, Caroline, departs quickly, waving cursorily at us all while breathlessly talking about a train to catch, elderly parents to get home to. Others stay to mingle.

When I get to my bus stop a quarter of an hour later, Caroline is still there, now really very anxious. She smiles at me in vague recognition, eyes darting towards the horizon of Commercial Road in vain. I commiserate, but then wonder whether I shouldn't encourage her to employ those two words we have spent the day immersing ourselves in. After all, there will be more trains, and her parents aren't going anywhere.

But then the universe suddenly realigns itself to our rhythm, as can sometimes happen, and coughs up a pleasant surprise. The bus arrives.

We exchange a smile of relief. 'Oh, thank fuck for that,' she says.

Like all of us, she's a work in progress.

Seventeen

One day, I am sent to interview a journalist like me, but a proper one, a war correspondent for television news. Out of a flak jacket, she is less serious and quick to laugh, wonderful company. She tells me about her time in Ramallah and Islamabad and Amman, and I am light-headed with envy. She agrees to answer what everybody always asks of people like her: what draws them to such dangerous territories? 'To tell the story,' she says, simply.

She shows a generous, and seemingly sincere, interest in my work, and I find myself telling her, as if in competition, of the only experience I have had that is comparable to her far more grown-up endeavours, a trip to Israel a few years ago for an American magazine, our hosts so keen to show us the unblemished tourist side of Tel Aviv that they went to laughable lengths to shield us from the reality of everyday life there. The photographer and I essentially spent an enforced seven days in its red-carpet five-star hotels and Michelin-starred restaurants, none of which were of much interest to the young and self-consciously adventurous demographic the magazine appealed to. If I wanted to see the truth, I'd have to hunt it out.

I tell her about the morning we were taken to a vibrant food market, accompanied by our guide and a chef who was going to cook us lunch from all the fresh produce we found there. We met eager stallholders, all of whom foisted upon us their wares – 'Special discount, my friend.' The chef, laden with fruit and vegetables and cuts of meat, saw an acquaintance coming his way, a locally famed sommelier to whom we were introduced; hands were shaken, backs enthusiastically slapped, tourists still a comparative rarity around these parts. But the sommelier was frowning.

'You should not be here today, I think,' he told us. 'I have a very bad feeling.' He looked nervously over either shoulder, a bad spy in a B-movie.

I asked him what he meant.

'Bomb,' he replied, explaining that there had been rumours of an attack here today, perhaps on the market itself, the perfect place for maximum casualties. (A bomb had exploded in a nearby falafel shop just two weeks before we arrived, killing two.) Our guide began remonstrating with the sommelier, telling him that he should not be putting the frighteners on a couple of journalists who were here to write nice things about their city for the good people of America. Potential tourists, in other words.

Our guide bustled us onwards, suggesting we leave the market anyway, to go and see the owner of a shop that made jewellery out of leather: necklaces, bracelets, even anklets. 'You can interview her. She is interesting.' I firmly suggested otherwise, insisting that it was my intention to write about the real Tel Aviv, not an airbrushed version.

'But this is not what we agreed,' he countered, threatening to talk to his boss, who would call my editor, who would then contact me to tell me off.

It was approaching midday, and the market was at its busiest. It was easy to give the guide the slip, to disappear down behind the fruit stalls, piles of empty cardboard boxes towering beside them. The guide didn't have my mobile number; we would be lost to him until we chose, finally, to return to the hotel.

Without him, a very different side of the city revealed itself. We submerged ourselves in the labyrinthine alleys of the market, a photo opportunity at every turn. The cafés we went to were cheap, rough and ready, full of life, the coffee black as tar. In one we spoke to some young women who told us that night-life started late in Tel Aviv, after nine. 'We stay in to watch the evening news to see if any bombs have gone off.' If there had been no explosions, they would get dressed up and go out; if there had been one, they would assess the severity, check to see if any of their friends had been casualties, and then would very likely go out drinking in another part of the city instead. 'It's life,' they said. 'We refuse to live in fear.'

In a park, where we shaded ourselves from a merciless sun, an elderly Hasidic Jew approached me with a concerned look on his face. He rested his hand on my arm and gazed into my face. I saw wisdom in his eyes. He told me that I had a big nose and that my fringe was too long. If I cut my hair short, it would take the attention away from the protuberance. Later, along the seafront, we were halted by police who had just found a suspect package on the beach and were in the process of cordoning off the area. We were the first to be stopped, a crowd gathering behind us, and so we were lucky: ringside seats.

The suspect package was a small backpack beside a beach towel. Even I could tell from my distant vantage point that it contained nothing more sinister than a pair of underpants, their owner having likely mistakenly left the shore without them, but this did not stop the dispatching of a small radio-controlled tank which puttered, gingerly and comically, across the sand towards it, stopping a few feet from it, then raising a protuberance of its own, something that it took me several moments to realise was a mini machine gun.

The crowd bristled, but nobody took a step back. Each of us wanted to see what happened next.

Even anticlimaxes can be thrilling. The policeman with the remote control in his hands lifted a thumb, then pressed on a button I felt sure must have been a bright shade of red. Though the tank was small, and its machine-gun arm comparatively tiny, the sound it made was impressive, the retort loud, echoing in my ears and the pit of my stomach. It fired four shots, paused, then fired a further two.

The bag did not explode. The policeman now approached with confidence, unzipped it and retrieved a posing pouch and a towel. The crowd duly dispersed, the road open again, business as usual until the next suspect package, the next quickly spread rumour.

'We drink because we can,' a group of friends told us later in a cavernous bar in the trendy Jaffa district, over fluorescent cocktails. 'And in defiance.'

On the way back to the hotel, late at night, we crossed a square where otherwise observant Jewish men, wedding bands on their fingers and clutching at their tzitzits, sought rough trade under the safety of darkness, creating Kama Sutra shadows that spilled from the bushes.

The morning after, over breakfast, the tour guide asked where we had gone yesterday. I told him about the bomb scare.

'I wish you had not seen that, and I hope you don't write about it,' he said. 'This is not typical of our country, you know.'

But it is, or at least it was. A week after our return, the food market we had visited did become a target. The rumours had been true. Many were injured.

'And so why did you stay at the time?' the TV news correspondent asked me now. 'Why didn't you leave when your tour guide told you to?'

I explained of my excitement at being able to witness how people lived their lives in compromised situations, and that I felt lucky to be able to tell their story. I had thought Tel Aviv a beautiful city, full of fascinating, resilient, complicated people. The inherent danger of living there was what made it so vivid. I hadn't wanted to leave.

'Then you are one of us,' she told me, a compliment more generous than she could have known, given that I was already fretting about how I would negotiate my fatigue on the long trek home.

As we said goodbye, she gave me her card, encouraging me to contact her. I told her I would, knowing full well I wouldn't, couldn't.

I brood over my conversation with the war correspondent for weeks, and realise that what I had said to her about witnessing how people lived their lives in compromised situations pretty much summed up how I was living my life now. My illness was a compromising one and had extinguished my sense of adventure, but not entirely. I wanted it back.

A few weeks later, and surely under her lingering influence, we rashly but entirely logically decide to move to China. The sense that life is out there while we merely paddle in its shallow end becomes increasingly insistent and painful. Elena is keen. We weigh up the pros and cons, more cons than pros, among them the conviction that the children, who crave only familiarity and friends, would never forgive us, and still decide it makes perfect sense. I act fast. I call up a local estate agent with a view to putting the house up for rent, and I cancel magazine subscriptions. We will go for six months, maybe more, but certainly not less. I buy books on the country, and pore over them in a frenzy of research.

I am raring to go. At night, we look at websites for international schools in Shanghai, comparing one against another. They are all prohibitively expensive, so we decide that while Elena works, making the money, I will homeschool the girls.

It seems like the most unhinged, lucid plan we have ever had.

There is some context here: my condition had made me a fantasist long before now. Three years previously, it was Bristol we were going to move to. The nightmare neighbours were still with us then, I was essentially housebound, and so Bristol offered an out. When in doubt about so much in life, flee. We'd been to

Bristol several times, and liked it. Bristol would do, even though neither of us ever really wanted to leave London.

Then, one morning, we read in a newspaper that Ho Chi Minh City was fast becoming a major international hub, increasingly popular with Western start-up types and youthful entrepreneurs. We fell into neither camp, but we had visited Ho Chi Minh once in our previous lives, and loved it so much that we were reluctant to leave. An idea, fully realised, instantaneously dawned: forget Bristol. We would go East!

It's always healthy to foster a lively dream life, but perhaps not when it spills over into the real one, consuming waking hours and sleepless nights. But when you are ill, or long-term unhealthy, dreams become a buoy on which to cling in the hope that it will float towards new horizons. And ours remained eminently tangible. If I could be tired in London, why not in another major international city? We decided to keep our options open, and considered Kuala Lumpur, Singapore, Bangkok – anywhere, as long as it was far, far away, and promised adventure, new leaves turned.

And then, one day, the planets align. Elena is sent to Shanghai for work, training scientists on how to achieve optimum lab results. China is an emerging, rapidly growing market, and a potentially lucrative one. Her boss wonders whether she might be prepared to travel to China multiple times over the next few years.

'It's a shame we don't have anyone based out there,' her boss says to her, and Elena does well to keep her voice free of the hysteria mounting within her when she replies, evenly, 'Yes, it is a shame.'

This, we reasonably conclude, is a sign. China works. Elena could get a secondment to Shanghai. We would follow her out there, and I could write, could correspond for magazines, newspapers.

She comes back from her first Shanghai trip in high spirits. Summoning the courage, she asks her boss about the likelihood of a six-month transfer to the city. It would be something for the CV, she says, and could work well for the team. Her boss likes the idea, and tries hard to make it work. For the next few weeks, it is all we talk about, a secret between the two of us until all is confirmed. The estate agent keeps calling, desperate to erect a To Let sign by our front gate. We monitor the daily pollution levels in Shanghai, and start shopping at the local Asian supermarket in preparation, noodles somehow a foreign concept to our girls, who insist they prefer spaghetti. Gradually, they come round.

But by the time Elena goes to Shanghai again, many long months later, the possibility of a transfer is abruptly off the table. Despite early positive signs, the Chinese cannot quite commit to the course her company offers, and so it simply wouldn't prove cost-effective.

And so, just like that, our dream is packed neatly away, its full ramifications to brood over defeatedly at a later date, and our world shrinks back into its usual parameters, leaving us thinking of what might have been while reverting back to the life we know, and leaving me with the new normal I am by now desperate to be shot of.

In the weeks and months following the Let Go seminar, I find myself muttering fuck it repeatedly, sometimes daily, aware now of tension, or anxiety, the moment it arises, and gradually transforming my inner 'no' into something approaching a 'yes'. I say it, and I slope my shoulders, exhale and let go. It helps. As does meditation, which is increasingly becoming both habit and ritual, something I do not even think about any more; I just do it. I am up and doing it before seven every morning, then fit in another session before picking up the girls from school mid-afternoon. And if I am out, on a bus, a train, then I close my book and close my eyes, and the world shrinks away. Slowly but steadily, my physical limitations are diminishing by stealth. I no longer bother keeping a diary.

I interview a bubbly TV celebrity, an American living in London, who tells me she too meditates, and in fact spends much of her downtime travelling the world's health retreats for days of silence, chanting, group hugging and introspection, as well as having her own daily routine at home. It turns out we both rise at the same time each morning to do it, though she does it arguably better, and more properly, in Lycra and in the lotus position in a room she tells me she has decorated specifically for the purpose. She tells me about balancing her chakras, and I nod knowledgeably, because I sense she wants me to, but already our connection is withering away. I do not balance my chakras.

I think I know what chakras are. They came up in previous meditation sessions, but I edited them out of my consciousness because it felt easy to do so. They are (I look them up later, for confirmation) the energy centres in our body through which energy flows, and there are seven of them: the root chakra, which represents our foundations and feelings of being grounded; the sacral chakra, which gives us the ability to accept others and be open to new experiences; the solar plexus chakra, which boosts confidence and self-control over our lives; the heart chakra, which gives us an ability to love; the throat chakra, for communication; the third eye chakra, which encourages us to see the bigger picture; and the crown chakra, which represents our ability to be fully connected spiritually.

I grasp the concept of them, ish, but what I cannot grasp is how to balance them, and what to do with them when I do. I ask her, the bubbly TV celebrity, and she tells me she simply focuses on them: 'I don't have to do anything else, just that. It's enough.'

I think that perhaps the chakras are beyond me, a little too Eastern and wholemeal. But this is fine. John C. Parkin would tell me to fuck it, of course, to do what I feel comfortable with for now, and no more, to take it one step at a time, to assimilate myself gradually. So I do.

Eighteen

It is about this time, by now over a full year into my adventures in alternative therapy, that I find myself craving a more straightforwardly psychoanalytical explanation for what I am doing here, this tireless, and slightly frenzied, pursuit for health by whatever means necessary. The answer, simply and fundamentally, is that I am searching for *help*: help in understanding my new self, and wanting, to some extent, to be looked after by someone, *anyone*, in the wake of the most dragging illness, and to have restored what has been so conspicuously lost. When we develop a long-term condition that forces a change in the way we live, it is nothing less than an assault on the very notion we have of our self. Where have we gone? Who are we now? To find a way back, we seek out guides, mentors, the loudest voices, proponents of affirmative action. In our search, we cast our nets wide.

'When you are ill without the benefit of a diagnosis that is of any use to you, then what are you supposed to do?' the psychoanalyst Susie Orbach will say to me. 'If you have been a person of action, and doing, then how do you do, and act, when you continue to feel so unwell for such a long time? It is a dreadful situation to be in, and so no wonder it's a struggle.'

To help process the struggle, I require now an educated overview into what my search might have left me with, and, pertinently, what I might have gained from it all. I want the opinion of someone I have heard of, with a public body of work behind them, respected in their field, boasting letters after their name. I am familiar with Susie Orbach's work, have read her and admired her, and found her radio series on theraphy illuminating. I decide she'll be ideal.

She grants my request for an interview, and we meet just once, for an hour. As suggested earlier, I have long been fascinated by psychoanalysts – their owl-like silences, the stealth of their attention spans – and Orbach doesn't disappoint. Curled up on a handsome leather armchair in her North-west London practice, she listens to my story with what strikes me as deeply professional acumen, all ears, barely a word spoken, appraising me not with judgement but with a cool and languid separation that, by the end of our hour together, convinces me she is half feline. I had been hoping, with habitual naivety, that she would do most of the talking, unfussily imparting psychological smarts, and that I would take notes. But she tells me that she doesn't know me, isn't familiar with my case, and so I have to talk first, and explain as much as I can in the time permitted. So I do. I expect her to rein me in from time to time, but she doesn't, and whenever we fall into what I instantaneously perceive to be an awkward silence, I fill it with more babble. On those occasions when she does talk, I immediately lean forward to better absorb her words, as if each were sap from a tree that I want to carefully collect and preserve.

'From what you've told me so far,' she says at one point, 'you've had some kind of serious breakdown within your system that was essentially crying out: *Help! I need help!* Now, I cannot possibly know yet what you did to break your system, but you clearly overstrained it, you became exhausted because of that, and so at some point you simply stopped.'

She asks me why I didn't seek out psychoanalysis in the first place, and I answer as honestly as I can: that, through my own ignorance and perhaps compounded by initial misdirection, I believed myself to be physically unwell, not psychologically. By the time I accepted that there was a psychological malfunction going on, I didn't know where to turn, or to whom. Frankly, I also didn't have the necessary capital for psychoanalysis. When I tell her about my failure in securing CBT, she tells me that CBT wouldn't have been the right kind of therapy anyway (the NHS, of course, suggests otherwise). 'It's not about meaning, it's about behaviour,' she says.

She believes the fact that I felt less tired – or, in her more psychoanalytical terminology, that I felt more *safe* – at home than I did outside suggests that my condition might well have had its roots in some kind of phobia. 'Maybe the journalist who was running around the world all the time simply needed to be home more?' She shrugs. 'But, look, I don't know. There are so many possible explanations for what happens to people, and people are all individual.'

Had we met when I first fell ill, she says, she would have striven to secure as much medical oversight as psychological, considerably more so than I myself had managed. 'If somebody is given your diagnosis, which is not really a concrete diagnosis at all, then I certainly wouldn't want to reduce it to the psychological. I would want to regularly liaise with a doctor – although,' she adds, 'that has already proved problematical for me in the past.'

Orbach had previously overseen the case of a colleague whose patient had chronic fatigue, but the patient's doctor, who had been treating her for the condition, wasn't happy that she was also in therapy. 'There were protocols, presumably, and as a result of these complicated protocols, she suffered. She went downhill fast, though she is getting better now. But that was really shocking to me. Usually, you cooperate as a therapist and a doctor. But clearly not in this case.'

Why?

She sighs. 'I wish I knew. I'm not used to this sort of competition between professionals. And I can't say I find it particularly helpful.'

I tell her about the alternative health practices I've dabbled in, my experiences with energy practitioners and meditation practitioners, those who try to eradicate my negative thought patterns by stopping them with repeated affirmations and reciting more positive ones; I tell her about the attempted kinesiology via pendulum over Skype. And while she makes it clear to me that she is no expert in the alternative market, which means that her opinion might be no more solid than anybody else's, some of it, she concedes, does sound a little unusual.

'Obviously, there are wonderful people out there who have found ways of helping people, but there are also those whose qualifications to practise might have come from a weekend course. In many ways, it's no different to a 12-step programme, a fellowship of hurt people who get better by helping other people. I don't have any particular problem with that – therapists have their own histories, after all – but it's how we use it, and under what circumstances.

'I confess I don't know very much about kinesiology, but the methodology you experienced, via Skype, is problematical for me. I would have thought that, even in terms of its own science, doing something over computers wouldn't work. What about the electricity between the two machines? I'm sorry, but the physics of it sounds crazy. I would think you'd have to be in the same room for it to work, even in the ways they suggest it works . . .'

As far as banishing negative thought patterns by announcing loudly, in my head, STOP!, she suggests that that also presents issues for psychoanalysts, 'because we are not trying to get rid of bad thoughts; we are trying to help people manage what they find difficult in life. So not to extract it, not to perform exorcisms, but to work *with* them.'

I explain that, as I had understood it, exorcism in this respect at least had become necessary, directly because my bad thoughts had become such harmful ones, and were limiting my health, and my life, accordingly.

'Yes, but bad and harmful thoughts are part of the human condition. When you go to a therapist, you try to understand what those harmful thoughts are a protection against, and learn how, in time, you can accept disappointment and hurt, rather than turning it into self-hatred. What we talk about is not leaving the bad thoughts behind but rather, through gradual understanding, changing that negative dynamic inside of you. It's more about finding that bit of you that can dare to be okay with yourself when you have been caught up in a very bad pattern. So our approach focuses on a different emphasis, ultimately.'

(Later, I go back and consult Anna from the Optimum Health Clinic about this. Might they be wrong, I wonder, to advocate such harsh neurological pattern breaks after all? Anna tells me that she understands where Orbach is coming from entirely. 'You don't want to make the bad bits wrong, you don't want to demonise any part of yourself, because that is to cut yourself off from it. And the negative thoughts are, in essence, just trying to protect you, which is why you ultimately do need to engage with them. But the problem, from a chronic fatigue perspective, is that this is quite a long process, and the idea of using stops, or equivalents, is simply to try, as quickly as possible, to calm the system down. If we just worked with you emotionally, then we would likely get to the same point, but that can take a really long time to do that. So while we are striving to get more clarity on what's going on emotionally, we are also trying to calm the system down as quickly as possible.')

Had I initially sought out a psychotherapist, Orbach says, they would have talked less and listened more. 'A therapist would have been interested in what this illness meant to you, how scared you were by it, what your feelings were, your history of work, your parents' history; the whole picture.'

And by simply talking about it, I ask, and coming to understand it, my physical symptoms – and the overriding fear I had of them – might have diminished, and I might have become better quicker?

'I think so, yes.'

I tell Susie Orbach, briefly, about the final two practices I underwent. The first, The Lightning Process, was another mind/body training programme, this one claiming success over all sorts of issues: anxiety, low self-esteem, panic attacks, eating disorders, depression, chronic pain, irritable bowel syndrome, multiple sclerosis, chronic fatigue. There was also much controversy surrounding The Lightning Process, but it does have that ultimate marker of approval in the 21st century: celebrity endorsement. Actors and sportsmen and women have done it, so too singers, explorers, the poorly children of celebrated TV presenters. According to testimonials, it has made them well again, cured.

It is run by a former osteopath, Phil Parker, who overcame his own difficulties in life – in his case, a bad cut that nearly severed his hand and that many doctors incorrectly believed would mean an end to his career – with an overwhelmingly positive mindset that simply refused to take on board any sort of negativity. He harnessed his self-belief and went on to achieve his goals, professional and otherwise (for someone with a bad hand injury, he plays a deft guitar). He now works to help others harness their own innate self-belief. I met with Phil Parker, and came away convinced that I have never encountered a more can-do person in my life. His optimism – distinctly not of the loon variety – was catching.

The fact that Parker was, like many of his peers, patient before practitioner is telling, says Susie Orbach. 'Maybe sometimes, when something works, there is a compulsive need to repeat it in order to reinforce their own experience of it. So by giving to others, they are also giving to themselves.'

Parker told me that the solution to conditions such as mine was to find a way to get our physiology reset, but in a positive way. The course he runs lasts three full days, and the gist of it is to discover how you can use your neurology to influence your health by developing self-coaching conversations with yourself and becoming immersed in empowering memories and expectations.

'The challenge of this sort of illness is to find a way to say that you are in control here, and as a result, to go about life in a different, more proactive way. The best person to access health for you,' he told me, 'is yourself. There is no drug that can do it as well. It is you that has to do the hard work, but the good news is that you are capable of it. We all are. We all have the same physiology, so if one person can do it, why can't everyone?'

I had heard similar sentiments before, of course, but there was something in the way Parker dispensed it that left me changed after the course. It became a mantra to go along with my other mantras, only this one stayed with me. Perhaps because he was a rarefied communicator, or perhaps I was simply ready, at last, to enforce some kind of lasting change. But while The Lightning Process didn't go on to cure me as quickly as its name likes to suggest – some of those testimonials claim rapid recovery – something did nevertheless alter within me, an audible clunk almost, the sound of me replacing one mindset with another, negative for affirmative at a stage in the illness where I thought I might never be affirmative again.

I then tell Susie Orbach about my final experiment, with hypnosis. I wasn't sure what I thought of hypnosis as a form of treatment, largely because hypnosis is mostly marketed, within the media at least, as a circus sideshow, something that makes good television when convincing willing audience members to cluck like chickens. I learned, however, that the world of science has taken hypnosis entirely seriously for some time now. The more we come to understand about the brain's plasticity and malleability – and the more direct influence we have over it – the more hypnosis comes to the fore. It is now being used as a treatment for all manner of conditions, chronic and otherwise. One definition for it, according to the Oxford English Dictionary online, describes it as 'an induction of a state of consciousness in which a person apparently loses the power of voluntary action that is highly responsive to suggestion or direction . . . Its use in therapy, typically to recover suppressed memories or to allow modification of behaviour, has been [recently] revived but is still controversial.'

As an alternative treatment, it is no more controversial than anything else I had done over the last few years, and no less. Despite it being used more and more as an adjunct of mainstream medicine, its practitioners still seem to use it primarily as a tool to help people lose weight, stop smoking, conquer their fear of flying, have better sex and better sleep. But in each instance the underlying objective is achieving greater communication between mind and body, developing a heightened persuasion, calming the cortisol and emphasising the power of self-belief.

I spoke to one hypnotist in New York who used it to delve into her patients' psychological problems. 'You don't really know what you're going to find,' she told me, which was why she urged me, in seeking a hypnotherapist for myself, to recognise the difference between hypnotism and hypnotherapy, and said that when seeking the latter as treatment, you should obtain it only from a licensed mental health professional.

'The subconscious mind has years of collective memories and behaviour to tap into, and let me tell you they are not always peaceful places,' she said. 'It could bring up all sorts of pain and distress that needs to be dealt with, and dealt with in the right way. We're talking issues here that may have been repressed, ignored, sometimes for a great many years. So what the hypnotherapist does is try to deal with them and put them back in a positive way.'

Tracking down a hypnotherapist who was also a licensed medical health professional wasn't as easy as I hoped it would be. Many didn't want to talk, and plenty didn't want me to write about them. One who did was unlicensed in this regard but was a Master Practitioner of Neurolinguistic Programming and a licensed hypnotherapy instructor. I'll call him Dave. His approach to treatment was to focus on a particular point in someone's life, an episode that might have left them scarred or traumatised, and then attempt to wipe the slate clean by revisiting that period via a timeline. Unlike in talk therapy, he didn't want the patient to identify the issue out loud, with a view to discussing it thoroughly, he merely wanted them to identify it privately for themselves.

Timelines are commonly used in hypnotherapy to help focus on the here and now, to overcome symptoms and to achieve freedom from blocks in pursuit of fulfilment and growth. Patients travel back through their own personal timelines, and stop off at an event that may be deeply embedded within their psyche. They address this episode and think about how it made them feel, then travel back up to the present day, having hopefully addressed the issue sufficiently to leave it in the past. This makes it all sound rather swift. While talk therapy can go on for months, if not years, Dave the hypnotherapist saw patients on average just three or four times. 'It works,' he told me.

Later, I read up on the use of timelines in this fashion and found that it is similar, but not identical, to Gestalt therapy, a form of psychotherapy that focuses on the individual's experience in the here and now, and that recognises that an individual's self-awareness can become impeded by negative thought patterns and behaviour. Its aim is to help people overcome the impediment.

A definition of it reads: 'A physical, biological, psychological or symbolic configuration or pattern of elements so unified as a whole that its properties cannot be derived from a simple summation of its parts.'

I do not even begin to understand this, of course, but what I do manage to glean is that Gestalt is much practised, and appears successful.

The first time Dave hypnotised me, he did so with such an absence of ceremony that I was unaware he had done much of anything. He simply asked me to sit back in my reclining chair, close my eyes, relax and be led by his guiding voice. A moment later, he was talking to my subconscious, and asking it to alight upon an event in my life that was in some way formative, a time of great stress or fear, for example, and establish when precisely this might have occurred. Was it, he asked, offering multiple-choice answers, between the ages of one and seven, during birth itself, or before birth? My first thought was: *Before birth? How does that work?*

I settled for between one and seven.

He did not want me to tell him what the episode was, but merely asked for words that might sum up my emotions at the time.

'Fear? Worry, possibly.'

'Good. And what else?'

I had to think more. 'Insecurity?'

'Insecurity. Good. What else?'

My mind was blank. I could not say anxiety because anxiety is merely a synonym for fear and worry, and I did not want to repeat myself. So I simply said, 'Um…?' But suddenly something came to me. 'Anger.'

'Anger. Good. What else?'

'Nothing,' I said. 'That'll do.'

Still addressing my subconscious, he asked me what, if I could go back to my seven-year-old self, I would say to him in order to reassure him, to mollify him. I felt self-conscious as I responded, 'That everything will be okay? That he shouldn't worry? He'll survive this. He'll get stronger.'

Dave pushed, gently, for more words, responding encouragingly to each one I managed to summon up. Now he ushered my subconscious back along the timeline to the present day, bringing with me those affirmations, that positive feeling.

Slowly, he brought me back into the room, whispering that I should open my eyes, but only when I felt good and ready to do so.

I opened them, and reached blindly for my glasses.

'Have a drink of water,' he said.

My first thought, while still blinking into the temperature-controlled gloom of the room, was: when is he going to hypnotise me? This was quickly followed by: is that it? There had been no hocus-pocus, no transformative effect. He said that he had spoken to my subconscious, but I felt fairly sure that it was my conscious mind that replied. But then how would I recognise otherwise? All I knew was that I felt entirely present in the room at all times. I had been aware of my bum on the seat, of the collar of my shirt annoyingly close to my chin, my feet flopping on the stool. While my thoughts had strayed carelessly to my bicycle chained up outside, and where I might stop off for lunch, was he really communicating with my seven-year-old self?

Eighteen months previously, Anna from the Optimum Health Clinic had suggested I had difficulty engaging with my emotions. I was too analytical, I asked too many questions, and was keeping my feelings at arm's length because that is what I had learned to do. Arm's length was safer.

Is this why I was still stuck?

The second time I saw Dave, I made a concerted effort to let go more, to really travel down that timeline and offer up my subconscious to him on a plate. I wanted to feel the emotions now. No more suppressing.

I am seven years old again, perhaps eight. Nine? We haven't moved into the house yet, and are still nine floors up in the tower block. It has been a strange night, my mother falling asleep on the sofa in front of the television, something I have never seen her do before. She had been in a foul mood during dinner, and so I am grateful, now, for the quiet, but also unnerved by it. She sleeps right through my bedtime; this is also unusual. I try to make noises to wake her, cough, turn the sound up on the television. She does not rouse. I wander into the kitchen and discover something else unusual: the sink is filled with dirty plates, not washed yet. My mother is fastidiously tidy; she always washes up immediately. The cold tap is trickling. It must have been trickling since dinner, which was hours ago. Now it is overflowing. Water is spilling slowly but steadily onto the floor. There is a blossoming puddle of it. What do I do? Something prevents me from reaching up and turning it off myself, from disrupting all the plates, the saucepans, from stepping into the puddle – perhaps because then I would be complicit. Instead, I must go and wake her and tell her, but I know she will be furious. Though I do not possess the comprehension at this age, I know at some instinctive level that sleep for her is escape from the wretchedness of her life right now. Her husband isn't here again. They are fighting when he is. Soon he will be gone. There is no money. We are alone. The last thing I want to do, then, is wake her up. I feel scared. I return to the living room and sit back down in front of the TV. I cough again, because if I wake her up by coughing, then this will be an accident, not my fault. I laugh a little too loudly at Benny Hill.

At some point she wakes. She looks confused. The cushion's pattern is imprinted on her cheek. 'What time is it?' she asks. She jumps up, tells me to go to bed, sees the state of the kitchen and shouts. I can hear tears in her voice.

Then, later – and I could be conflating evenings here, or it could be the same one – I am lying wide awake in bed. I can hear my mother in the kitchen, proper tears now. At some point my father comes home. There is an argument, raised voices, slammed doors. He's gone. Memory is an unreliable thing, but I seem to remember thinking: go, good riddance. We are better off without you. But my mother's tears I do not like. They make me want to rush to her, to try to comfort her, to tell her it will all be okay, that I am still here. I hope she will be all right, that in the morning things will be better in that undefined way things sometimes are at the start of a new day.

But now I start thinking about her dying. If she does, what then? Losing a parent is one thing; losing both would be careless. I try to imagine what life might be like alone, without her, and how badly I would miss her. It is a horrible thought, but I revel in it. I make myself cry. The pillow is wet, and I feel small and vulnerable, and scared. I cry for a while, but then I get bored of crying, and I think of good things instead: Steve Coppell on right wing, Sammy McIlroy on the left, the goals of Jimmy Greenhoff. Eventually, I fall asleep.

To the hypnotherapist now, I offered many of the same words I had offered him the first time around: don't worry, it will be okay, I'm with you, I'll look after you. All this will make you stronger.

He brought me round again, and we chatted for a while, and then I went. And that was it, no more. Presumably, then, I left

Dave with my slate clean, able at last to move on with life. Or at least that was the idea. I found myself hoping it had worked.

But it had all seemed suspiciously easy. I'd been expecting something harder.

When I ask Susie Orbach whether the hypnotherapy might really have worked in some crucial way, her response is deliberately ambivalent. 'I don't know,' she tells me. Her honesty, I confess, intrigues me: in the world of alternative health, I have been used to promises, a great many of them boastful ones. There is a lot of convincing that goes on among alternative therapists, many of them as confident, as bullish, as Kanye West. But in more mainstream health practices, nobody promises anything.

Then she says, 'Look, perhaps it did help, and if it did, then why not? What I would say, from a psychoanalytical perspective, is that it might have worked in some way because you felt guilty about the relief that your father left, and about feeling pleased that you could co-parent even though you were clearly burdened by it. The hypnosis might have helped you feel better about that. But then this, to me, is just another form of exorcism, and what I would want to know is: to what end? I'm not saying I want people to live endlessly through guilt and horror and conflict, but the question here is: how do we manage to live with these things in our lives rather than sever ourselves from them?'

She asks me if I feel my experiences this past year have worked, and if so, with which therapy, and why. I tell her that I like to think that they have all worked, cumulatively, each in their own way. And even with those that I didn't get very much from, I still came away with the conviction that more is possible than I might have otherwise realised, that I am more in control of my fate, my health. They have each helped encourage me to take responsibility for myself, to know how to calm myself, to say fuck it, to centre myself, not merely to say yes instead of no but to *feel* it – to feel *yes* – in mind and body alike.

And if they have worked for me to some extent, I ask her now, then why have they? How?

'Maybe you simply got curious about yourself rather than remained merely curious about the people you write about in your work? And maybe because you had such a shock that this happened to you, you have finally learned to have a more compassionate relationship with yourself? Does that sound possible?'

I say that I thought I already had a pretty compassionate relationship with myself.

'But, you see, we are not brought up to think about ourselves in "self" terms. We are brought up to be productive. You were productive. Your curiosities, as a journalist, were outwardly directed. The arrogance of our Western traditions is that we think we know everything about ourselves, when really we don't know very much at all. So much of what concerns us is unconscious.' She laughs. 'All you have to do is try marijuana or acid once to know that we really don't know so much of what is going on inside our heads, right? There is a conceit that we are full of self-knowledge, but it is only a conceit, I'm afraid.'

More and more of us, she believes, are looking towards alternative practices these days, and the reason for that is rampant capitalism. Because we now have our basic needs covered – food, shelter – this has freed us up to focus on the smaller things in life, things that previously might not have concerned us at all. So we are self-centred more, we seek perfection, acceptance. Our cravings have gone up the wall. We feel increased guilt, envy, that we are in some way insufficient, lacking. And all of this builds stress, and the stress compounds.

'It's very hard for people today to be brought up to have massive ambition, and live in a consumer society in which they have to brand themselves constantly. If you are poor, it is completely impossible to belong. I feel that we have moved from a society of contribution to a society of display, and that it is very difficult for people to find their own place within it.'

To the point where it can make people unwell?

'Yes,' she says.

Psychoanalysis, she insists, doesn't offer a magic bullet. 'But it does offer a methodology, and it offers you the capacity to reflect, to think and feel about yourself. If you had sought out a therapist when you first became ill, you might have been prompted more to listen to yourself, and to discover within you what it is that has been a problem. That's a very different form of practice to the ones you've been going through, but I do believe it could have been a very effective one.

'I don't want to be an evangelist for suggesting that mental pain is good for people,' she continues, 'but I do think that, when it comes, people can either grow from it or sink under it. There is so much human suffering out there, and so little provision for cultural discourse about it that is of any use whatsoever. There is also not very much help within our existing health service, or in our education system, in terms of offering people a way to understand and cope. So when you do get something like a phobic response, as you did, you often don't have a chance to use it to understand and grow.'

Which is why, for so many of us, long-term illnesses and conditions can leave scorch marks. 'Yes,' says Susie Orbach, 'but they may turn out to be very good scorch marks in the end.'

I expect her to say more here, to fill her economical sentence the way I would – with more words, and yet more words – but she doesn't. Instead she does that endlessly enigmatic psychoanalyst thing of allowing her gaze to simply settle on me, forcing me not just to respond to what she has said, but to *think* on it. And I do. For days and days afterwards, I think on what she said, and relive our conversation time and again, looking, I think, for clues and answers and direction and implied wisdom. I come away with two things: many more questions, and the conclusion, late as I come to all conclusions in life, that therapy can be highly nutritious.

I should have had more of it.

Nineteen

The morning I learn that I don't have chronic fatigue after all is a curiously anticlimactic one. I'm at an NHS hospital that looks spectacularly old and unloved, even by NHS standards. It is so conspicuously empty, of both doctors and patients, and so sadly downtrodden (paint peels from walls filled with notices for long-passed events; footprints echo down its worn-out linoleum corridors), that I half wonder whether this hasn't actually been closed down years ago and I am only really here in a mischievous dream full of psychological hints that point to my state of mind. I am the only person in the cavernous waiting room, and while I wait, in sinister silence, I browse a 2011 copy of *Chat* magazine. Unsettlingly, I find that my phone has no service. I'm in a windowless twilight zone.

I'm here because of Professor Peter White, the specialist consultant who was quick to tell me, when we met a few months previously, that this area of illness was rife with misdiagnoses and contradiction. He had told me that four out of 10 cases of CFS are misdiagnosed by doctors and immunologists. 'So if you are not given the right diagnosis, it's no surprise when the treatment they offer doesn't work,' he had said.

I had met him to talk about his work rather than to ask for medical advice, but as we parted he kindly offered some. He said that I should look up my old friend Dr Dolittle, and request now to attend one of the CBT courses he had initially recommended. 'I'd ask you to come on one of mine,' Professor White added, 'but you live too far away from here, and the NHS doesn't work that way. You have to approach your local service.' He said it would be useful for me, and that I would definitely qualify this time. After all, it had been Dolittle himself who had suggested I attend his clinic in the first place, specifically for graded exercise therapy, but he had also mentioned their CBT classes, back then an unknown acronym to me; he could hardly reject me now.

When, several weeks later, I receive a letter from Dolittle's office rejecting my request – I still don't meet the criteria – he does offer, as an ameliorative perhaps, an appointment with one of the clinic's doctors to talk through any issues I might be struggling with. Three months later, and here I am in the forgotten suburban hospital, two long bus journeys from my home but still deemed 'local', quite possibly in a waking dream of my own imagining.

The doctor I see, at least, is lovely, a kindly, sympathetic woman in her mid-30s who talks to me for an uninterrupted hour, her questions more thorough than any I have been asked at any point in the last three years. Her conclusion, she says, is definitive: I don't have chronic fatigue. Of all the symptoms they look out for in such cases, the only one I possess is the fatigue itself. I show no signs of depression; I remain mentally alert. Yes, I experience torturously long periods of extreme tiredness, but there is no brain fog, no aversion to bright light or loud sound. Essentially, I function fairly well.

She goes on to say that post-viral fatigue is a little more vague. It is possible that my persistent fatigue is more physical in nature than mental, a problem with my T-cell regeneration not functioning as it should. But this is a theory they are still awaiting concrete evidence for.

'Anyway,' she says, 'discard everything you have heard for the last three years.'

I am more than a little bewildered.

Dr Dolittle had himself, of course, suggested after our 10-minute consultation that I was merely 'post-viral', though he did concede that the fatigue itself was clearly, in the literal sense at least, chronic, and the course of treatment he recommended was the same course he recommended for those suffering from CFS and ME. Consequently, everything I subsequently pursued was as a result of that consultation, and geared towards those with fully diagnosed CFS. I wonder aloud now, to the doctor in front of me, why he did that. Why recommend me for something he would ultimately bar my entry to?

She smiles uneasily. 'I don't know.'

What she does tell me is that while my condition has clearly been, and still continues to be, debilitating, it is less serious than the other kind, less restricting in the long term, and so I should probably try to dismantle the unhelpful mindset Dolittle had unwittingly lumbered me with, and instead take this latest diagnosis with the optimism it deserves. 'It's good news,' she says.

In the 1983 film *Trading Places* starring Eddie Murphy there is a scene towards the beginning in which Murphy is begging for money on the unfriendly streets of Manhattan. He is sitting on a wooden crate on wheels, his legs concealed beneath him, dark glasses hiding his eyes. The suggestion is that he is a war veteran, blind and legless, a tragic figure deserving of charity. But the police, wise to the ruse, apprehend him. They remove his sunglasses, then lift him up out of the crate until gradually Murphy is forced to lower the legs he still possesses. Desperate now, he feigns surprise, then jubilation.

'I can see! I can see!' Murphy cries. Then: 'I have legs! I can walk! Praise Jesus!'

This scene comes back to me as I leave the hospital this morning. I have just been told, essentially, that everything I know is wrong, and with it a tacit suggestion that had I been given a longer initial consultation, then things might have played out differently. Yes, I would still have been ill, but perhaps without Dolittle's 'worst-case scenario' I would have reacted with less fear; my brain would not have quite reached catastrophe; the fallout would have been less.

It is raining steadily now, and as I am crossing the road, the bus, *my* bus, passes in front of me. There is still some distance to the bus stop, and under normal circumstances I would let it go on without me. It's only 20 minutes until the next one. But seeing as I don't have chronic fatigue, I make a mad run for it. After all, I have legs, I can walk. Praise Jesus.

I make it, coughing and wheezing, my heart a basketball against my ribcage. I wheeze all the way home as I wonder what I should do with this new information, how it impacts me, what difference it makes, and should make. What do I care whether it's called 'post-viral' or 'chronic'? There is no straightforward treatment for the former anyway, so the latter was always my ultimate destination. Either way, that single symptom – fatigue – has been a permanent resident of my recent life, and a defining part of it. Friends tell me I should be furious, and those irate CFS forums I never visit would probably encourage me to start sending letters of complaint, death threats.

But what would anger buy me? The fact is, my condition – and my reaction to it – is nobody's fault, not even my own. We have a health system that is really pretty amazing, and that success-fully fixes most people when they are most clearly broken. But not all of us can be easily fixed. Those who fall in between fall in between. We are complicated creatures, after all, and experts say that modern life is making us more complicated still.

Besides, I have by now come round to my new reality. I don't welcome it, I don't willingly accept it, but it's here, and I'm getting through it. We all adapt, all the time, and for all different reasons. And that's what I've done. I've adapted, even if I have lost certain things in the process. The thing I truly lament is that my children might never know the old me, the me who never sat still, who never stopped *doing* things. But then our children never really know the old us, do they? They don't need to. They settle for what they have. In this particular case, they settle for a father mostly sitting in a succession of comfortable chairs. Only I feel the contrast, the before, the after.

It's the hare and the tortoise. It's life. Best get on with it. And anyway, I have tools now, tools that come in handy in unforeseen ways, helping me deal with the stresses – and occasional all-out panics – of everyday life.

There are a particularly stressful few days I go through with work, in which some people I interview express subsequent disappointment at the article for not being quite the hagiography their team had hoped for, but rather a more honest assessment of their high life and times. To compound this, there is the suggestion I may have some of my facts wrong. With this comes the unspoken threat of legal action.

Though I have never knowingly written a puff piece, and would never want to, it is rarely pleasant to know that something of mine has caused distress, even if that distress is ultimately generated by some very sensitive egos that should know better. There are lots of emails from their people, containing lots of exclamation marks, and I react to each of them poorly. This is compounded by a late-night phone call on a Saturday from their LA-based management further expressing their many disappointments. I apologise for any unwitting offence caused, but defend my right to produce a balanced piece. 'But the fans didn't like it,' I'm told. The more she talks, the more my ribcage knits itself together. My skull becomes uncomfortably tight. Saliva evaporates from my mouth entirely, and working my tongue around the words I need to continue my defence requires a lot of concentration.

The night is disrupted, dreams contaminated. The same negative thoughts spiral around my head, and I reach for The Lightning Process's mantra to break them. It works. I sleep. In the morning, I meditate for longer than normal, and though I have no concrete idea whether it helps, I can see that it is possible the stress might have been worse had I not. Either way, I'm glad I can turn to these things, these skills, instinctively.

It takes a good while to revert to normal. The emails cease, and the implied legal threat recedes when it emerges that I did not have my facts wrong after all; the offended party simply had a selective memory. In the time it takes me to fully unknot, I overanalyse my reaction despite the fact that overanalysis is the last thing I should be doing, a pointless, energy-sapping exercise. But it is hard not to, because the longer the stress lingers, the more I fear I might crash into another bout of debilitating fatigue. I am damaged goods, after all, and can no longer afford to expect to have the instinctive ability to brush it all off.

The debilitating fatigue never quite arrives, but while the stress lingers, I am fearful it will, and consequently am hardly fuelled with vitality. Instead, I am comprehensively tired, which is just another way of saying fatigued, thus providing me with the last link in what essentially is a self-fulfilling prophecy. It's a murky place, my head.

Whenever I find myself in such a spiral, I go over these pages, to remind me of the methodology, the psychology, the pick-me-ups, and all the solid, sound advice pointing to ways out. I frequently recall the telephone conversation I had with a fellow sufferer a few years back, the man it was recommended I talk to as he was further along his path to recovery than I was, but who told me, when we spoke, that emotionally he was reeling. Of course he was, and I realise why now. It is easy to forget good advice when we most need it, when we crash and panic and flail, which is why it is so necessary, for me at least, to turn back to it and read it off the page as many times as required. It's my therapist, perpetually on call, saying the same old things because that is precisely what I need to hear.

Occasionally, then, I catastrophise. But these are blips, and blips pass. I can, and do, moan that life is all effort these days, but life always was. The goals just feel richer now, and in my less am-dram moments, I realise that as a result of my efforts and, more pertinently, the teachings of others, I really am at last improving, I am at last getting better.

The irony that the overriding symptom of these fatigue-related conditions is a slowing down of things just when the signs of ageing were cruelly speeding up was not lost on me. And so while I was looking elsewhere, I appear to have fallen head-first into middle age. It didn't even announce its arrival. If I had had the time a few years ago to anticipate it, I might have expected incremental changes, the gradual physical announcements of one bodily ache and pain after another. Instead, it's as if it has happened all at once. I have gone from a comparatively healthy 42-year-old convinced he was still in the first few vigorous toilet flushes of second youth to an abruptly older gentleman. The bodily aches and pains quite possibly have nothing to do with any lingering fatigue as much as they do with my body beginning to go to pieces, as bodies my age tend gradually to do. I work in maintenance now.

Though I do not deliberately look for evidence that I am not the only one – safety in numbers – I nevertheless find it everywhere. I come across a report on the news one morning that says Britons are the unfittest people in the Western world, that none of us do very much exercise at all. We tend now towards indolence, and do nothing but sit around all day, at home, at our desks. Group activity comprises watching television together. If we have to travel anywhere, we do so by car or public transport.

The result is an increase in heart disease, diabetes, obesity and early death. This means that with the exception, perhaps, of avid dog walkers, our collective energy levels are fast dwindling as we become increasingly habituated to our lack of collective motion. Fatigue might just be a byword these days that could apply to anyone. Must get dog.

I read a travelogue, Tim Parks' *Italian Ways*, in which the author says he can chart his own ageing process in terms of the energy he still has to tackle stairs. At one point he is late for a soon-departing train, and so has to hurry. But he is a man in his 50s. Hurrying no longer comes easy. He struggles.

'At 35 I could do the steps two at a time from the metro platform to the ticket hall and again from the ticket hall to the platform – a total of five floors, I'd say,' he writes, '. . . arriving at my train bathed in sweat but barely panting. At 40 I was panting hard but still forcing myself. At 45 I was obliged to take the top section just one step at a time and still feared my legs might buckle under me or my heart burst. I would collapse into my seat with pulse thumping and a taste of blood in my throat.'

From other people's limitations we draw comfort. I too am the same with stairs now, and have to prepare myself for them both mentally and physically. I used to skip up them without effort, always carelessly. Shortly before becoming ill, for instance, my right foot misjudged one of the steps at home, the nail of my big toe snagging upon it and lifting free from its secure moorings, then resettling in a pool of blood I can still see today. I no longer snag toenails; I'm too slow for that. It takes me impatient time to climb them today, but I still reach my destination because my destination is going nowhere.

I have come to accept this as just another unavoidable sign of the inevitable toll of my ageing, and nothing more sinister than that.

One morning, I Skype with an American who, after several personal life crises, renounced what he believed to be a prescriptive 9-to-5 existence in favour of living more spiritually, and more wholly for himself. He moved to Hawaii, became a Taoist and now helps guide those struggling through midlife via, he says, 'a system of faith, attitude and practices set towards living your inner natural life rather than what others try to shape you into.'

We speak for what seems like hours but is surely significantly less, and it is at the point at which he suggests that, were I to follow his lead, I might be lucky enough to live until I am 120 that I wonder quite what it is I am doing here, now, conversing with him. He had requested we speak mid-evening his time, which is early morning for me, and so I am up in my room, with the door closed, as a family breakfast unfolds without me downstairs. I am having trouble following the man's line of thought, unsurprising giving my thorough ignorance in the wisdom of Tao, and I begin to glaze over at much of what he says, then catch myself and worry that I am wasting both his time and mine.

With the kind of clarity that only ever occurs a little too late, I realise that I should now stop moving from one would-be guru to another, and that perhaps my plan of trying to write myself better has reached its natural conclusion. The state of being ill long term is curiously addictive. You become victim to it, sensitive to its mood swings. It can be difficult not to fall into its trough, and spend the rest of your life seeking wisdom from people who claim to have seen the light. But as the Hawaii resident talks I start to feel that it is time to get back to living my life, complicated as it still is, and push to the margins what has for too long now been centre stage.

'Bodily decline is the story you have been taught because you have been taught that you have two halves to your life,' I hear him saying. 'Work, then retirement. The longevity techniques in Taoism teach you to learn to live more gracefully with your age. Not all people age visibly. You need to learn to pace yourself without stress, and in a way that is sustainable. Do that, and the body can go on great for years and years and years.'

But I have absolutely no intention of living until I am 120; the next few years alone should keep me busy enough, a period in which, if I am to improve my situation, I will have to do so by myself, alone. I tell myself that I need to get out there and participate in the everyday, and that the more I do so, the more the fear that has gripped me will gradually recede. This at least is my hope. And though I don't know it yet, this will more or less come to pass. I will in time become more mobile, and will resume an outdoor life. I shall take holidays again, and fly to those destinations like everyone else, navigating vast check-in halls and far-flung departure gates that take forever to walk to. I shall go on beach holidays with my family. I shall hire a motorbike in Greece and disappear into the mountains on winding, empty roads, screaming euphorically into the hot winds at the sense of giddy freedom I thought I would never experience again, and I will come back home so desperate to recreate that situation that I will buy a motorbike – and all the gear, and take the road test, and secure insurance – within a few hyper-manic days of my return that will prompt me, briefly and metaphorically, to crash. I shall give in to the girls' three-year pleadings and get them the dog they always wanted, and I will walk it in the sun and the wind and the rain, *me*, the man who couldn't walk to the corner shop and back this time last year now getting reacquainted with London's beautifully rambling parks, barely able to believe that it is me with a lead in my hand, and that the dog at the end of it is mine. And, yes, I will continue frequently to battle with bouts of excessive tiredness that lay me low for days, but I will win the successive battles painstakingly, one by one by one.

For now, though, the Hawaiian Tao master is still telling me about the negative stories I have been taught about how life is supposed to progress. I wrap things up, wishing him goodnight, and I go back downstairs to the story of mine.

In the drawn-out moments that it takes me this morning to roll over and squint at the alarm clock, I realise that it is a weekday. Tuesday. The school run looms. But first, my routine.

I groan, get up, scratch, yawn and feel my age. This is all no less brutal now than it was a year ago, and it still requires discipline to climb up out of bed and away from it, but I do it, and my complaints dissolve by the time I reach the shower. I have long since dispatched with my Hour of Power. There are only so many movies you can run in your head until you have seen them all. So instead, post-shower, I do 10 minutes of yoga, which I perform assiduously but not, I fear, in any way yogically. I remain at a constant level with yoga, and this despite the fact that earlier this year I took a 10-week course in it. The course was for beginners, the hope being we would graduate into something other. Advanced, perhaps. But I do not seem to have a body made for advanced yoga. Beginner is my limit.

Then it's down to breakfast. No toast any more, no coffee, but porridge, recommended for its slow-release-energy properties, into which I sprinkle mulchy flaxseeds and a squirt of agave. The kitchen is full now of tell-tale signs of our joint sustained health kick, because Elena works in maintenance too. One cupboard is full of oatcakes, to my mind the only food-stuff that makes flaxseeds exciting. Another has brown rice, pulses. The dark chocolate, contraband these days but tasting better than ever, is hidden (and frequently replenished), but the fruit bowl is proudly displayed, and always heaving, the fridge full of vegetables. We juice now, too. Everybody does, it seems.

With the children gone, safely delivered to their classrooms, I return home to work. My approach here has changed, too, in some small but intrinsic way. I still love the job, and I am still at my desk before nine each morning, eager to start, to fill the screen with words. But somewhere over last few years I have ceased pushing myself quite so hard, with such fervent mania. This hasn't been easy. But giving up that incessant drive to bag commission after commission as if life depended on it (which it still sort of does) has been, undeniably, a blessed relief. I can breathe now.

And if there is less work for me today, then there is for everyone. My trade is changing, a new generation emerging, new ways of doing old things, Instagram far more important than words, tweets preferred to a long read. And that's fine, I'm fine with it. Really. Except that – no, no, I'm not, of course I'm not. I'm furious, livid at the prospect of my imminent extinction. But then perhaps I must simply try now to reposition myself elsewhere. After all, our greatest glory is not in never falling, but in rising every time we fall. Confucius said that.

My own personal enlightenment stretches only so far. I am still, for now – who knows, possibly forever – stuck in my story, impervious to my true essence. But I am working on it, a solid plod in what I trust is the right direction. I do not want all of this to have been in vain. I want to learn from it, to come out of it a better person, to myself if to nobody else.

I have tried a mere handful of the hundreds of alternative therapies out there, all of which boast their own convincing salesmen and women, many of whom have come through considerable tribulations of their own, in some cases defying science. These are the extraordinary people. I conclude that I might be one of the ordinary ones, because while I am certainly getting better, slowly but defiantly, there has been no great epiphany for me, no Damascene conversion into new light, no overnight miracle.

Instead, I have ingested as much as I could. I have understood some of it, got confused by a lot, and have likely already forgotten much along the way. I am still unpicking all the unhelpful behavioural traits that landed me in this mess in the first place, and I am forever on the lookout for signs of progress.

It is demanding work. Much of it requires a complete overhaul. But then I am in midlife, and habits die hard. I like a lot of my habits, even the bad ones. They make me *me*. Leaving them behind will be a wrench.

Two jobs today. I meet a singer mourning the loss of his father from dementia, and an actor who has spent many decades attempting to get to grips with depression. Yet more lives being put together again.

Then it's to the modern equivalent of a greasy spoon for a bread-free, nutrient-rich lunch, something very likely on a bed of what I'm told is quinoa, and then back on the bike, over the bridge, to the train station. The first half of Waterloo Bridge is a slight incline, a slog, so I pedal hard. But it is worth it, because on either side I am surrounded by my very favourite city view: the Gherkin, the Eye, St Paul's, the Cheese Grater, the other one. It was this I missed most, this view, when I was stuck at home all the time, wondering if I would ever get to see it again. It is sunny, and warm for September, the wind in my hair. London is looking radiantly proud of itself.

I reach the best bit now, the halfway point, and the beginning of the descent. My bike picks up pace. I overtake a bus and several other cyclists. As I approach the IMAX cinema, I look to my right and see what I had hoped to see: nothing, no cars, no traffic. I don't have to brake. My wheels are going too fast now to pedal any faster, and so I careen at effortless speed around the roundabout, leaning into the bend. On my left, a car appears out of nowhere, fast, rudely encroaching into my lane. It cuts in front, I swerve, and a second later I am alongside it. I look in to see a pretty young woman driving, oblivious to me. Next to her, in the passenger seat, is a man peering at his BlackBerry, thumbs flying across its keys. He looks up, and I look back into the face of Alan Yentob. This fact is of more interest to me than it is to him, because he already knows he's Alan Yentob. He casually disregards me in favour of returning to his email. Ahead, the looming traffic lights have changed from green to amber. Both me and Alan, and his driver, cruise on through as it changes to red. I need to leave him now, and take a sharp left towards the station.

It is uphill from here, all the way to my platform, but I'm still going at such a clip that I need exert no energy at all. I take my feet off the pedals, weaving in and out of pedestrians with what passes, for me, as wild abandon, the wind still in my hair, and for a sustained moment it feels as if I could go along like this for ever, uphill but effortless, prepared for whatever comes next.

But only for a moment, because then the hill becomes too steep and the bike slows. I start pedalling again.

Epilogue

I have always liked stories, a good narrative with its beginnings, its middles and ends. You can read them like a book, and I suppose I am all the more invested in this one because this one's end – here, these last few pages – might just represent my having got fully better. Unfortunately, that hasn't happened yet, not entirely, and I am beginning to accept that it might never.

What is *better*, anyway? My old self? My old self, the healthy one, is seven years younger than the me of today, seven years fitter, and still in the ignorant bliss of comparative rude health. He hasn't had a psychological fallout from which he is still trying to put the pieces back together, and so my old self has likely gone for good, replaced by the new me. But I'm better than I ever dared hope. Two years on from my adventures in alternative health, I still tire easily, I still subconsciously impose limitations on my physical activity, and I still crash intermittently. But I have my life back, a variation of it at least, and I'm relieved, and grateful. Perhaps, then, this is as good as it gets? And perhaps, as Susie Orbach told me, the scorch marks I bring along with me might just turn out to be good ones.

'For me, it was very transformative,' says one person I speak to who went through a similar experience. 'There were so many benefits, in so many ways, to my having been ill, because positive things have come out of it. We learn from it, and we can grow; life can become fuller as a result. I know that may be difficult to hear about if you are still in the midst of it, but I've had many conversations with many people about this. Initially, they focus on what they've lost because they can no longer be the person they had been before, but there is also a dawning of recognition, the fact that perhaps they weren't as happy as they could have been. So, yes, sure, you do lose certain things, and I have, but you gain other things, among them a real appreciation of life. You start to value the simple things, and you form a much greater connection to what is really important.'

This message, for all its hackneyed intent, remains an alluring one: from illness comes wisdom. It is an angle I am well aware of, having reported on such stories for the past 20 years via interviews with many people, often very successful women and men, the surprising majority of whom have, in their own pursuit of a career and success and happiness, sometimes catastrophically burned out along the way, and have been forced into living in newly sustainable ways: the pop and rock stars with their pill addictions, their therapies and NA meetings; the singers with Crohn's disease and depression; the fearless but fragile American artist with bipolar disorder who eventually found a cure, after 30 years of searching, via yet another developing alternative practice, this one called EMDR (Eye Movement Desensitisation and Reprocessing), which sounds bizarre but is said to be effective in the treatment of trauma.

'There is nothing wrong with me now at all any more,' she told me, offering a low-wattage smile when I had been expecting floodlights. Then she added: 'Which is sort of a problem in itself.'

I met someone recently, a former pop star, who had lost several decades to drink and drugs, his wife left him, and he ended up in his 50s in rehab, depressed and alienated and utterly lost. So he became newly spiritually ravenous. 'Who am I?' he wanted to know. His search, ongoing, is all-encompassing. He has joined the Masons. He practises Transcendental Meditation, and reads books by Jesuit priests, the verse of Sufi poets. He has undergone shamanic interventions and ayahuasca ceremonies, craving higher states of consciousness and a better understanding – of everything. Death looms somewhere on the horizon, and he wants to reach that particular conclusion clearer, repentant, humble, at peace with his shortcomings, and better prepared to navigate, soberly, what remains.

'Know thyself, you know?' he said, only slightly tongue in cheek, hailing as he does from Camden, not California. 'Life is a journey. Learn. Absorb the useful, disregard the rest. And when you seek something and you find it, know it, own it.' I asked him if he was happy now, if happiness was what happened to people who read Sufi poetry. 'I'm content,' he replied. 'I've learned that there is strength in vulnerability, that vulnerability is a powerful thing. Don't be afraid to show yours. You know, there is a lot going on right now, in us, in the world. We are in a crisis time, we've lost sight of one another, our true hearts. We need to be part of the paradigm shift from the age of capitalism to the age of consciousness. We have to wake up, to be aware, and we have to share that awareness.'

'We change in fundamental ways every seven to nine years,' the Hawaiian Tao master had told me. This was news to me. I must have coasted ignorantly through my previous changes, but I am all too aware of this most recent one. And he's right: it has changed me in fundamental ways. I have lost confidence but developed a certain survivor-like steel. I have learned to pace myself and even, for moments at a time, to fully switch off. I am slower, calmer, more present. I am less fraught, less frenzied. More resilient. I walk, don't run, in every sense. Life may feel more effortful now, but only because I am so assiduously aware of its constituent parts. Often, this brings reward.

From time to time, I try to pinpoint any positives to glean from all this. When I compare life before with life after, the former wins in almost all categories. I miss living off an endless energy resource, and a part of me is still affronted by the fact that it proved not to be endless after all. But then again it's good to stop running in all directions all of the time. I still meditate, though not always as rigorously as I should, and my yoga routine is less about the breath than it is about simple stretches. In other words, I could do better, but the intent remains. I'm unfit but active, ish; there's room for improvement. If I look hard enough, I see that life is indeed now full of endless daily miracles, mostly of the humdrum kind, but which I cling to because I know how much they have cost me. I have saved a small fortune in shoes. My marriage, I think, is stronger, and I am lucky to have an amazing wife who took the 'in sickness and in health' bit seriously. I must work to repay this. I am watching my children grow up, because I'm a very present father – too present, the girls might argue, because I am always here, never anywhere else. But I want to be here with them. Nowhere else is quite as much fun.

Being ill has paid off in other ways, too. I have met some truly fascinating people, people I can learn from, and write about. Fascinating people to write about is all any writer craves. They have taught me more in the past three years than I have learned in the previous 30. I hope to retain at least some of their teachings.

And I have come, grudgingly, to accept that I am Jack Lemmon in *The Odd Couple* when all I ever wanted to be was Walter Matthau. This, perhaps, is my fate.

There are worse.

ACKNOWLEDGEMENTS

Many people gave me a lot of their time during the writing and researching of this book. I would like to thank each of them, but particularly: Will Williams, Anna Duschinsky, Phil Parker, Alex Howard, Susie Orbach, Professor Peter White and Elaine Hilides. Thanks also to Julie Clark, for unstinting friendship. To Natania Jansz, for key creative counsel. To A.L. Kennedy, Cathy Rentzenbrink and Meg Rosoff, for such generous and encouraging words. I am enormously grateful to the whole team at Bloomsbury, particularly my editor, Sarah Skipper, and my wonderful publisher, Charlotte Croft, who made it all happen, and steered the book – and me – so capably. I'd like to thank my beautiful daughters, Amaya and Evie, vital life forces who kept me sane, and kept me focused. Mostly, I would like to thank my wife, Elena, who did nothing less than help make me well again when I was convinced that getting well again might never happen. She was my doctor, my nurse, my support system, and she was so incredibly kind. She is my best friend, my foil, and my very favourite feminist.